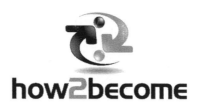

how2become

How to become a
BEAUTY THERAPIST

www.How2Become.com

D0318471

Orders: Please contact How2become Ltd, Suite 2, 50 Churchill Square Business Centre, Kings Hill, Kent ME19 4YU.

You can order through Amazon.co.uk under ISBN 978-1-910602-21-8, via the website www.How2Become.com or through Gardners.com.

ISBN: 978-1-910602-21-8

First published in 2015 by How2become Ltd.

Typeset for How2become Ltd by Anton Pshinka.

Printed in Great Britain for How2become Ltd by: CMP (uk) Limited, Poole, Dorset.

Disclaimer

Every effort has been made to ensure that the information contained within this guide is accurate at the time of publication. How2become Ltd are not responsible for anyone failing any part of any selection process as a result of the information contained within this guide. How2become Ltd and their authors cannot accept any responsibility for any errors or omissions within this guide, however caused. No responsibility for loss or damage occasioned by any person acting, or refraining from action, as a result of the material in this publication can be accepted by How2become Ltd.

The information within this guide does not represent the views of any third party service or organisation.

CONTENTS

INTRODUCTION

How to Become a Beauty Therapist

Welcome to 'How2Become: The insider's guide to becoming a beauty therapist'. This book has been designed to help guide you through the steps to becoming a beauty therapist. By the end of this book you will have a full understanding of the beauty industry, what it takes to work within a salon and even how to start your own mobile beauty therapy business. Using insider information, we will provide you with the best interview tips and tricks, show you how to better your treatment procedures and help you to guarantee customer satisfaction. With the help of our experts, you will get a fantastic insight into the daily routine of a qualified therapist.

The UK beauty industry is currently worth £17 billion, and is set to rise substantially over the forthcoming years. The industry was one of the few areas not to take a hit during the recession. From 2008-2013, retail sales skyrocketed from £6.1 billion to £7.1 billion. With images of celebrities, beauty and style being broadcast to global audiences on a daily basis, people want a quick fix. The industry itself is ageless. Young people want to look young for as long as possible, and older people are trying to prevent ageing. As an aspiring beauty therapist, you are entering a hugely competitive industry, particularly if you have ambitions to open your own salon, or teach beauty at college level. Therefore, it is essential that you are prepared with as much information as possible, in order to give you an edge over your competitors within the field.

This guide has been split into useful sections, to make it easier for you to understand the different routes to becoming a beauty therapist. Using the advice of qualified professionals, we will take you through college and apprenticeship application, salon work, mobile beauty therapy and other available options. We will teach you how to tailor your CV to gain employment at an established salon, and the types of activity you will be expected to perform within each sector.

With the right work, and perseverance, you can become a highly successful and talented beautician. This book will show you how. We are confident you will find it a useful resource in your pursuit to becoming a beauty therapist.

CHAPTER 1

Why should I become a beauty therapist?

As a beauty therapist, your primary objective is to make your customers look and feel the best they can. As the statistics show, beauty is a growing industry. A customer will only return if they feel you have provided them with the most comfortable and most reliable treatment available, but ultimately they will return. No product is constant, and that is why the beauty industry has maintained its level of success over the past few years. People want, and need, to look and feel good about themselves, and helping your customers to achieve this can be a highly rewarding process. Both men and women can be extremely sensitive about their looks, and therefore it is your job as a beauty therapist to reassure and make them feel comfortable.

Amongst beauty therapists, it is almost universally agreed that the most important quality you must possess is the ability to communicate effectively with your customers. As we will see, even in college applications; an enthusiastic, interested and warm personality will give you an edge over those who might have more experience than you, but lack the right persona. Ultimately, beauty therapy is a customer service based field, and will bring you into contact with many different types of people. The salon should be a place where customers can relax, and even open up to their therapist. If you are someone who loves to meet and interact with people, and make them feel good about themselves, then this role is perfect for you.

As an anatomy based career, the work is always changing. You need not worry that you will be stuck performing the same procedures day-in, day-out. New developments and treatments are introduced every year, and this keeps the work fresh and exciting. As a qualified beautician, you will be required to adapt and learn these new techniques, making each year different from the last. If you are someone that ultimately decides to specialise in a particular area, there are many different routes you can choose. You can work in a salon, in the entertainment or modelling industry, become self-employed or perform door to door services. You will learn secrets about skincare, health and exercise that will not only benefit your clients, but yourself. If you are someone who desires to look glamorous and young, then working in an environment where you can learn about and gain access to the best treatments available, can only be advantageous.

As with every career, there are challenges. Beauty therapy is at times a physically demanding role, particularly when it comes to treatments such as massage. You will need to maintain high levels of concentration for several hours at a time, in order to ensure that procedures such as pedicures or manicures are performed to the best standard. You must also be completely comfortable with touching certain areas of the human body. Pedicures, back massages and Brazilian waxes are all a regular feature of every beauty therapist's day, and at times some of your customers may not arrive in the cleanest, or ideal, condition. You must possess the ability to work through these difficulties and perform the procedure regardless, whilst remaining as upbeat and social with the customer as possible.

Another challenge you might face as a beauty therapist, is customer demand. As stated, due to the influence of the media, many people have unrealistic expectations as to exactly what a session in the salon can do for them. You are of course qualified to advise and guide them on what you think the best procedure for them might be, but you must be prepared for clients who will go their own way regardless. Often, you may feel that the treatment you advised would have been more successful, but it it is important not to think of yourself as an artist in these situations, simply a service provider. This is where you can best utilise your customer service skills, either to convince the client to take the procedure you have advised, or in assuring them that what they have chosen has worked out for the best. If, in rare instances, the customer is angry or upset with the result of the treatment, you will need to use these skills to calm them down. In some cases, where a treatment has failed or gone wrong, the salon may offer the client a replacement procedure in order to correct the mistake. As a beautician, you should go into each day with a knowledge of when you will see each client, how long you have to perform the treatment and how long your breaks are in between. A replacement treatment will eat into this time, and therefore it is important to organise your time effectively, inform future clients that their treatment may be delayed, or subtract time from your own scheduled breaks.

Whilst writing this book, we interviewed a variety of experts within the field. You will find their helpful tips, on everything from manicures to customer service, scattered throughout this guide. We asked one of them what she thinks about the social benefits of the role:

'It is a personable job by nature, you have lots of really pleasant interactions and great conversations, and can learn a lot from the public! It can be relaxing to perform certain treatments, and you quickly learn how to handle and make people feel at ease.'

By now you are probably wondering, how do I get started in this industry? Here at How2Become, we will provide you with an in depth answer to this question. Most people who decide to take beauty therapy, do so immediately at the conclusion of their GCSE exam results. However, there are also a great number of candidates who decide to switch careers later on their professional life, to pursue beauty. While you will still have the option to train either via college or as an apprentice, there are also fast-track training providers available. These will cost you a small fee, but get you up to speed quicker than if you chose any of the former options. You will receive a Level 2, or Level 3 certificate from these training courses, exactly the same as you would from an apprenticeship or college course. In the following chapters, we will explore both salon and apprenticeship work, what they entail and how to gain a place on each.

CHAPTER 2

College Application

When enrolling for a place on a college beauty course, there are many things to consider. Generally, colleges look at your predicted grades, and base their decision, prior to the results themselves, on this information. The majority of colleges use an online admission system, whereby your application will be immediately passed on to the beauty department of that college. To help you decide which college you should apply for, it is advised that you either go into the college, or visit their website. There you will be able to find and download a full prospectus for the year ahead.

Each course uses a learning based module system. The VTCT awarding body decides upon which modules will be made mandatory, and then the college itself chooses from a range of optional modules. All current courses require candidates to have at the very least a C in GCSE English and a C in GCSE Maths. If you do not possess these grades, then you will be required to take classes in the subject, at the college you are applying for. These classes will run alongside the beauty modules, and will often be taught by the beauty lecturers themselves.

The Application:

Generally, if you are applying for a college, you should expect a similar form to this-

Full name:

DOB:

Gender:

Title: Mr/Mrs/etc

Ethnicity:

Prior Attainment Level:

Are you a British Citizen:

Have you been a resident of the UK/EU for 3 years?

Are you, or have you ever been in local authority care?

Do you have any unspent criminal convictions?

Address:

Postcode:

You will then be given a question in regards to your interest in the subject, and enthusiasm for the course. This is the most important part of the application. Here at How2Become we have prepared a sample response, which you can use as a basis for your own.

The question might look something like this:

'Tell us why you should be given a place on the course you have chosen, and why we should consider you for the course. You should outline your career ambitions, personal interests and any work experience, including voluntary work:'

A question such as this is looking for a number of different things from the answerer. The key word here is 'you'. The course administrators are clearly looking for a quality that sets you apart from other applicants. While they will obviously be accepting a number of different applicants, the emphasis in answering this question should be upon your own strengths, and how they can be applied to this course. You, the reader of this book, already have a distinct advantage in that we have already prepared you with the knowledge of what qualities a beauty therapist requires. As we covered in the previous chapter, you should be:

- Social and comfortable with people
- Enthusiastic
- Conscious of your appearance
- Willing to adapt and learn new methods and treatments.

This question also enquires as to the nature of your career ambitions, personal interests and work experience. It is a good idea in this case, to set your industry ambitions high. By telling the course providers that it is your future aim to set up your own salon, teach beauty or specialise at a higher level, you are letting them know that you are an applicant with a dedicated and enthusiastic attitude to the course, who will work hard to achieve good results. A lack of answer to this question will serve as an immediate red flag to the department. They are looking for interested and ambitious candidates who will go on to represent the college at a later level. You should therefore tailor your answer towards higher ambitions within the field. If you have relevant educational experience, particularly English and Maths, it would also be extremely useful to mention this.

In terms of both personal interests, and work experience, you should also take the same, positive approach. If you are someone with a lack of direct work experience, then it is okay to use indirect, or unpaid experience. For example, you may have spent many hours applying makeup to friends or family, or even cleansing your own skin. As we have highlighted, the most important quality that a beauty therapist must have is an approachable and friendly persona. If you can demonstrate this, it will help your chances. Any customer service related job will fulfil this requirement, or any occasion when in your personal life you may have had to deal with an angry or unhappy individual. The college are far more likely to proceed with your application if they see that you are someone who already possesses the personal qualities needed to succeed within the field. Likewise, you should tailor your personal interests towards what the course is looking for. Ideally, this should be a short one or two sentences, demonstrating that you are a social person, with an interest in beauty and helping people.

Using all of the above information, write out your answer to this question below, and see how it compares with our sample response, on the next page:

Tell us why you should be given a place on the course you have chosen, and why we should consider you for the course. You should outline your career ambitions, personal interests and any work experience, including voluntary work:

Sample Response

Dear Sir/Madam,

I am writing to apply for a place on your 'Level 2 Diploma in beauty therapy' course. I feel that I would make an ideal candidate, and possess the qualities needed to succeed within the field. As an aspiring beauty therapist, I am shortly due to take my GCSE's, and following these studies, would love to embark upon this course.

I am a social, outgoing person who loves to meet new people, adapt and better myself. I have future ambitions to either open my own salon, or teach beauty to younger people. I have always been meticulous about my own appearance, and frequently spend time helping both my younger sister, and friends, to perfect their own hair, make-up and nails. By the end of the summer, I will have achieved GCSE's in English and Maths, and am now looking to pick up the valuable tools and experience needed to work within the beauty industry. I believe your course, and college, are the best place for me to learn, and I would be very grateful if you could consider my application.

Yours sincerely,

As you can see, we have put ourselves across as someone who is extremely interested in the industry. This enthusiasm will draw the readers attention, and hopefully lead to a further interview.

In some college application forms, you may be asked 3 or 4 questions. Below we have listed some of the further questions you might expect to see, and included sample responses to each of them.

'Describe a situation where you have worked with people who are different from you in relation to age, background or gender.'

This question has been designed to assess your ability to work with others, regardless of their background, age or gender. Many organisations, especially those in the Public Sector, will want to see evidence of where you have already worked with people of different ages, sex, sexual orientation, backgrounds, cultures and religious beliefs. Remember to be specific in your response, relating it to a particular situation. Do not be generic in your response. An example of a generic response would be – 'I am comfortable working with people from different backgrounds and have done this on many occasions'. This type of response is not specific and does not relate to a particular situation.

Using the above information, write out your answer in the box provided, and then compare it with the sample response below.

Describe a situation where you have worked with people who are different from you in relation to age, background or gender.

Sample Response: 'Whilst working in my current role as a sales assistant I was tasked with working with a new member of the team. The lady had just started working with us and was unfamiliar with the role. She was from a different background and appeared to be very nervous. I tried to comfort her and told her that I was there to support her through her first few working days and help her get her feet under the table. I fully understood how she must have felt. It was important that I supported her and helped her through her first few days at work. We are there to help each other regardless of age, background or gender. As a result of my actions the lady settled into work well and is now very happy in her role. We have been working together for 3 months and have built up a close professional and personal relationship.'

Describe a situation where you have worked closely with other people as part of a team.

The ability to build working relationships with your colleagues is very important. Never underestimate how important teamwork is in an organisation. This question is designed to see whether you have the ability to fulfil that role. Remember again to be specific about a particular situation and avoid the pitfall of being too generic. Try to think of a situation when you have worked as part of a team, maybe to achieve a common goal or task.

Using the above information, write your answer in the box provided, and then compare it with the sample response below.

Describe a situation where you have worked closely with other people as part of a team.

Sample Response: 'I recently volunteered to work with a new member of our team at work. The task required us to successfully complete a stock take of the entire warehouse within a short time-frame. The reason why I volunteered for the task is because I am a conscientious person who enjoys working with other people, and carrying out tasks to a high standard. Initially I showed the new team member how to stock take in a professional manner in accordance with company guidelines. He had never carried out this type of work before and I wanted to ensure he was comfortable with the task, and that he was doing it correctly. Once I had achieved this we both then set about methodically working through each aisle, stocktaking as we went along. Periodically we would stop to ensure that the task was being done correctly. At the end of the specified timeframe we had completed the stock take and were able to provide accurate figures to our line manager. Whilst working as a team member I always concentrate on effective communication, focusing on the task in hand and providing support to team members who require assistance.'

Describe a situation where you have had to remain calm and controlled in a stressful situation.

When responding to this question, think of an occasion where you have had to stay calm and in control. This does not necessarily have to be in a work situation but it may be during leisure time or at home. Be careful not to answer this question generically. Focus on a particular situation that you encountered recently.

Using the above information, write your answer in the box provided and then compare it with the sample response below.

Describe a situation where you have had to remain calm and controlled in a stressful situation.

Sample Response: 'Whilst driving home from work I came across a road accident. I parked safely and went over to see if I could help. An elderly lady was in one of the cars suffering from shock. I remained calm and dialled 999 asking for the Police and Ambulance services.

Once I had done this I then gave basic First Aid to the lady and ensured that the scene was safe. The reason for taking this course of action was simply because when I arrived people were starting to panic so I knew that somebody needed to take control of the situation. By remaining calm and confident I was able to get help for the lady. As a result of my actions the emergency services soon arrived and the lady was taken to hospital. The Police then took some details of my actions and thanked me for my calm approach and for making the scene safe.'

CHAPTER 3

College Interview

If your application is successful, you will then be invited to an interview with one of the senior teaching staff at the college.

The first thing you will be required to do, is to fill in a questionnaire. Similarly to the original application, this will test your prior knowledge of the beauty industry, and your enthusiasm for the course. We have tracked down a sample questionnaire, and provided sample responses to each question, to aid you in your preparation for this process.

Sample Questionnaire

Please answer the following questions as clearly as possible:

1. Do you have any medical issues, or medical history that we should know about?

Always ensure you are honest with the institution, as this question is asked for your welfare/benefit.

2. What hobbies/interests do you have?

Similarly to the way we answered the initial application form, here you should tailor your answer to the question. Show an interest in the subject, but keep your answer short and succinct.

'I am very interested in hair, makeup and beauty, and often spend time helping my friends and family to perfect their own. I am a very social, outgoing person who loves to meet and interact with new people.'

How to become a Beauty Therapist

3. Why have you chosen beauty as a career?

Likewise with the above question, we can refer back to the initial application form. This is a great chance for you to tell the institution about your plans and future ambitions, and let them know how much you care about the subject. Once again, keep your answer short, succinct and on topic.

'I feel beauty is the ideal career for me. I have always been a people person, and a job that allows me to help and meet with new clients and customers on a daily basis is extremely appealing. I am some-one who cares deeply about the value of personal appearance, and in future, would love to use the valuable skills I will learn from this course, when working either in a salon or independently. It is my ultimate ambition to open a salon of my own, or teach beauty to younger people.'

4. What is the most important skill needed to work within this industry?

- Communication skills
- Dancing skills
- Singing skills
- Athletic skills

Answer: Communication Skills.

5. Why is it essential that you communicate effectively with clients?

- To have a chat
- To ensure they receive the correct and safest treatment
- To find out what they did at the weekend

Answer: To ensure they receive the correct and safest treatment .

As we have elaborated on, communicational ability is the single most important quality that a beautician must possess. Good communicational ability will help you to:

- Promote and sell products
- Keep the client relaxed
- Gel and get along with the range of different people you will meet
- Make sure you get all the information needed, to ensure the client receives the correct treatment.
- Ensure the client returns for another treatment.

6. Why is good personal presentation essential in the field of beauty?

This question is asking you to display a knowledge of the effect that physical beauty, and personal hygiene, can have upon clients.

'As a beautician, it is important that you hold yourself to the same values with which you would treat your customers. This is especially relevant within a salon environment, where you will be dealing face to face with customers. If a customer is being treated by a therapist who is well presented, clean and smells nice, then they are more likely to feel that said therapist can deliver the same results to them. They are also more likely to return for further treatment'.

7. Give two examples of good service, and two examples of bad service, when working in a beauty salon:

Good:

Bad:

This is a harder question, which requires a prior knowledge of the industry. Luckily, here at How2Become, we have already provided you with numerous examples of the type of work that you will be involved in if you get a job in the industry. Below we have listed a number of different answers to this question, for both good and bad.

Good:

- *Welcoming the client as they arrive at the salon.*

- *Taking the clients coat as they come into the salon.*

- *Engaging the client in conversation while they wait for their treatment to begin, and during treatment.*

- *Ensuring that you have logged and identified all of the correct information before starting a treatment, and making sure that the client understands everything that will take place.*

- *Ensuring that the work station is clean, hygienic and safe according to industry standards.*

- *Ensuring that you are well presented, hygienic and fit to begin treatment.*

- *Offering the client a drink/biscuit/food while they wait for treatment to begin, or during treatment.*

- *Ensuring the client is comfortable before beginning the treatment.*

- *After finishing the treatment, making sure the client is happy with the initial result of the treatment.*

- *Safe and friendly exchange of fee between customer and client, encourage or promote future products and purchases.*

- *Seeing the client out, fetching their coat, etc.*

Bad:

- *Failure to welcome the client upon arrival at the salon.*

- *If client has to wait, failing to inform them of how long they should expect to wait.*

- *Failing to offer the client a drink, upon arrival or during treatment.*

- *Failure to gain the correct information from the client before starting procedure.*

- *Failure to sanitise the work station and tools prior to treatment.*

- *Failure to inform the client of what the procedure will be.*

- *Failure to ensure the client is comfortable before beginning treatment.*

- *Failure to engage customer in conversation, resulting in a frosty, uncomfortable atmosphere.*

- *Failure to check whether the customer is happy with the initial result of procedure following treatment.*

- *Failure to see client out, exchange fee or encourage them to return next time. This includes a lack of product promotion.*

8. Are you someone who enjoys working alone, or do you prefer to work as part of a team?

This is another difficult question. In a question such as this, it is best to try and keep your answer as positive as possible, and highlight the benefits of both. As a beauty therapist, there will be times when you will be working both alone, and as part of a team. Your treatments will largely be a solo effort, but in ensuring correct and proper care of the salon, you will have to work effectively as a group. Remember that this is a people based career, so even when you are working alone, you will still be coupled with a client. If you have any relevant work experience, both alone or as part of a team, it is a good idea to mention it here.

'I am someone who enjoys the benefits of working both alone, and as part of a team. I love meeting new people, but it is on a one to one basis that I most excel. I am a fantastic conversationalist, and have been told that people often relax in my company. Therefore, working alone, one to one with a client, is an ideal environment for me. Despite this, I also value the group mentality of teamwork, and appreciate the necessity that collaboration between team members requires. Due to my warm, friendly and hard-working personality, I would make an efficient and capable addition to your team.'

Any relevant solo or team experience should now be inserted, along with an example of how you contributed/were important, to said team.

'During my time at my local fast food restaurant, I frequently worked as a team member. I had to ensure that I was in sync with the rest of the team, to establish fast and efficient production of food. Duties as a team member included: Helping other team members to reach their targets, making sure my own production was up to necessary speed, plus training and assisting new team members with the workload. During night shifts at the restaurant, I also completed a large amount of solo work, due to understaffing. I have successfully managed one half of the backroom by myself, and feel confident I could do the same in a similar environment.'

In some cases you may be required to take a comprehension exercise. This is to test your attention to detail, particularly when it comes to logging down the specifications of certain clients, and finding the right course of treatment. Below is one such example.

9. **'Congested skin is often painful for the sufferer.'** As the pores become blocked, the texture feels coarse, uncomfortable and lumpy. White heads and black heads will develop, along with a hardening of the epidermis over the pores, preventing sebum and sweat from reaching the surface of the skin.

Causes of congested skin:

- *Inadequate cleansing methods: old makeup and dirt builds up.*
- *Use of products that can clog up pores.*
- *Ill health. Toxins can build up under the skin.*

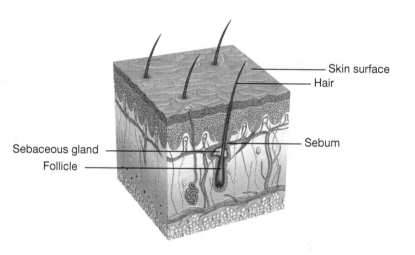

Now answer the following questions -

1. What is the texture of congested skin?

2. What can develop as a result of congested skin?

3. What effect does the hardening of the epidermis have?

4. Name two causes of congested skin.

Answers

1. The texture of congested skin is coarse and lumpy.

2. As a result of congested skin, white heads and black heads can develop.

3. The hardening of the epidermis prevents sebum and sweat from reaching the surface of the skin.

4. Inadequate cleansing methods/use of products that can clog pores/ill health-toxins.

Upon completion of this test, you will then be required to pass a verbal interview with one of the lecturers. During this interview, you will be judged on:

*   Appearance
*   Oral expression
*   Written expression
*   Enthusiasm
*   Personal hygiene
*   Language

Here at How2Become, we have tracked down a number of potential interview questions that you could be asked at this stage of the process. This is also fantastic practice, as many of the questions you may be asked will likely be similar to those asked if you applied to work at an actual beauty salon. If you perfect your answers here, you will have a much easier time gaining work in the industry when your course has finished. We have included direct interview tips at the end of this chapter, and during Chapter 5 and 6 of this guide.

1. Do you know what the course entails?

If you are someone who has done their research prior to the interview, then you should have no problem with this question. By showing the interviewer that you have researched the course and understand what it will involve, you are also showing them that you are an interested and enthusiastic student.

'Yes, I picked up a prospectus prior to this interview. I know that this course involves health and safety, product promotion, manicure, pedicure and massage techniques. I am particularly excited about the latter, as I am considering specialising in massage when I have completed the training.'

2. Why do you want to take the course?

As we have elaborated upon in the previous chapter, the interviewer here is looking for a clear and concise idea of what aspects of beauty the candidate is particularly interested in, and a rough outline of their future ambitions. There is nothing worse than saying 'I don't know' in an interview, as this tells the interviewer that you aren't interested in the course, and don't care much about the subject. Don't be scared to sound ambitious, the college want people who are eager and willing to learn.

'I would love a place on this course because I think it is the best way to prepare me for a future as a qualified beauty therapist. I'm really interested to learn more about massage techniques and skin therapy, and hope to apply these someday when working in a salon. I'm hoping to study all the way up to Level 3, and begin training with treatments such as Electrolysis.'

3. What makes you a good candidate for this course?

This is a question you should expect to hear in every interview. It is also a great question for you, because it allows you to sell yourself to the asker. By now, from reading this book, you should have a pretty good idea of what qualities a professional beauty therapist needs. You should tailor these qualities into your answer, and make yourself sound perfect for the course. While you should try to come across as confident and enthusiastic, don't be afraid to flatter the institution a little either.

'I am not just a great candidate for this course, but as a beauty therapist in general. I am a really social, friendly, outgoing person who loves to meet new people, and help them to feel good about themselves. I've always loved helping people; friends and relatives with their hair and makeup and now I'd love the opportunity to test these skills in the workplace. I still have a great deal to learn however, and this course will really benefit me in that respect. I really believe this college is the best place for me to learn.'

4. Tell me about yourself.

This is similar to the last question, but often this particular question is an attempt by the asker to get to know whether your personality is the right fit for the industry. Particularly in beauty therapy, personality is extremely important, and therefore you should treat this question as an extension of the previous.

'I'm very friendly and hard-working. I've got two younger sisters and have spent many hours helping them to do their hair and makeup, and teaching them to do it on their own. My Mum taught me when I was younger, so I've really enjoyed the experience of passing down my skills. On weekdays I work at my local fast food restaurant, and this has shown me lots about working as part of a team, and as an individual. But now I'd like to do something I'm really interested in; I love meeting new people and learning new things, so beauty is the perfect course for me.'

Before your interview, practice using the mirror at home. Make sure that you are able to put your answers across clearly and slowly. Many people talk too fast in interview situations, due to nerves. Remember that the most important thing in this interview is that the interviewer sees you as a friendly, social and interested candidate. It is extremely rare that college applicants are rejected from courses such as beauty, so just be yourself and you have a high chance of getting accepted.

We asked one of our experts, who regularly interviews candidates for the college she teaches at, what she looks for in an applicant:

'When conducting an interview for my college, the qualities I most look for in a candidate are: a personable and friendly nature, examples of what they have achieved, a sensitive and caring manner, ambition and drive. These are all qualities that I would love to instil on my students, to prepare them for life as a beauty therapist. Anyone who already possesses and can display them, immediately has an advantage.'

CHAPTER 4

Taking the course

According to your GCSE results, you will be sorted into 2 possible categories:

Level 1 Diploma in Beauty

Requirements: 5 GCSE's, D to F or equivalent.

Level 1 Beauty is a very basic programme, which mainly involves assisting, with less studied content. Candidates will learn and assist with basic skills such as application of day makeup, basic facial and basic manicure. This generally doesn't involve pedicure, advanced makeup, eye treatment or waxing. This may, of course, vary from college to college. Candidates good enough to progress will move onto Level 2 in the following year.

Level 2 Diploma in Beauty

Requirements: 5 GCSE'S, D's and above.

Level 2 Beauty is a regular programme that involves more content than Level 1, and less assisting. Candidates will learn and assist with everything included in Level 1, to a more advanced level, and this will also involve pedicure, advanced makeup, eye treatment and waxing. You will learn about removing unwanted facial and body hair, spray tanning, eyebrow alteration and skin cleansing. Similar to Level 1, this may vary from college to college. Since this is the level that the majority of candidates generally enter the course at, candidates are advised to check with their college if they wish for a full outline of the curriculum.

Following the completion of Level 2, candidates who are strong enough will move onto Level 3. This level can only be reached with both high results and attendance during Level 2. Level 3 is an advanced programme that involves more content than either Level 1 or Level 2, and more individual treatment work. This can include regular massage, Indian head massage, aromatherapy, electro therapy, non-surgical skin improvement treatments, and hot-stone treatments.

Each level counts as a standalone qualification, with candidates who are good enough staying on to move up to the next level. Your progress will be determined by both observational and online assessments, and your attendance over the course of the year. The observational tests will usually take place at the end of each module, and will decide 50% of your grade. The final, online assessment will decide the other 50%. You will be tested in areas such as:

- Health and Safety
- Product Promotion
- Treatment Procedure
- Customer Care

For most courses, you should expect the activity to be divided into modules. You will spend time learning a module, and then at tthe end of this module, you will be tested via a practical exam. The modules will consist of anatomical study, muscles, bones, the science of beauty therapy and actual practical work. Students should be aware that they will be expected to volunteer for each other as models to practice treatment on. For your observational exams, you will have the choice of bringing in a friend or member of your family to act as your treatment model. If this cannot be arranged, most colleges will have a list of willing participants who they can bring in to fulfil this role. These practical exams are decided on a pass or fail basis.

Here we have listed some of the most common practical modules, and what you would be expected to demonstrate in order to pass. We have also helpfully included some sample exam questions, which will give you a better understanding of the type of information you will be expected to learn from these modules.

Level 2 Modules

Here are some of the modules you might expect to take if you enrol in Level 2 Beauty. These can vary from college to college.

Healthy and Safety

This is one of the most important, and fundamental modules that you will take. You should expect to see this module on every college curriculum. Unlike most of the below examples, the observation for this module will be judged both via a separate module, and during the other practical assessments. This is to demonstrate, alongside your other practical skills, that you have the ability to work with the utmost care and regard for both you and your clients welfare.

In this module you will be expected to demonstrate:

* An excellent understanding of risk awareness.
* An excellent knowledge of how to reduce risks in the workplace.
* An excellent knowledge of how to deal with workplace hazards.

These conditions are situational and largely apply to the test which you will be taking. The module itself will deal with standard risk awareness in the workplace, such as fire hazards, chemicals, electricity, slips trips and falls. As you will be working in the cosmetic industry, safety with chemicals will be a particular point of focus.

Sales and Promotion

In this module you will be expected to demonstrate an ability to sell products to customers within the salon environment. For many salons, the ability to promote and sell these products is the difference between surviving and not surviving in the competitive world. Therefore, as a beauty therapist, is it crucial that you can demonstrate and possess the skillset required to do this.

Some of the things you might be required to demonstrate are:

- A detailed knowledge of salon products and services.

- An ability to identify products and services that may interest potential clients.

- An ability to correctly identify opportunities for promoting products and services to customers.

Facial Skin Care Treatment

In this module you would be expected to demonstrate an ability to perform procedures including: skin exfoliation, facial massage and mask treatments. You must be able to identify the correct procedure for the correct client, according to their skin type or condition. This module focuses heavily upon health, safety and hygiene standards.

As this is a module where you would be required to perform treatment, we have broken down some of the expected requirements needed to pass this module, into 'Before', 'During' and 'After' treatment.

Before treatment:

- Ensuring the work station meets the necessary treatment and hygiene standards.

- Ensuring tools and equipment are clean using the correct cleaning procedures.

- Identifying that the procedure chosen is correct for the client, and poses no threat to their skin or general health, by establishing their current skin care routine and taking a log of their responses.

During treatment:

- Using products and equipment according to the manufacturers' instructions.

- Using the correct exfoliation methods, ensuring maximum comfort for the client and clean, smooth skin.

- Using a clean and safe method of black and white head extraction, ensuring maximum comfort for the client and no damage to the skin.

- Learning and adapting massage techniques according to the needs of the client.

After treatment:

- Ensuring the skin is moisturised and client is comfortable following masking treatment.

- Ensuring the client is happy with the initial results and has knowledge of the correct aftercare procedure.

- Ensuring work station is left in a suitable condition for later treatment.

Eyebrow and Eyelash Enhancement

In this module you would be expected to demonstrate an ability to perform procedures such as eyebrow shaping, artificial lash treatment and eyebrow tinting. You must be able to identify the correct procedure for the correct client, according to skin tone or needs. This module focuses heavily upon health, safety and hygiene standards.

As this is a module where you would be required to perform treatment, we have broken down some of the expected requirements needed to pass this module, into 'Before', 'During' and 'After' treatment.

Before treatment:

- Consulting with client and logging details to determine the correct treatment plan.

- Performing a sensitivity test on an area of the client's skin, according to industry practice requirements, and recording immediate results.

- Explaining the treatment procedure to the client and ensuring they are happy to continue.

During treatment:

Eyebrow shaping-

- Cleansing and preparing eyebrow area prior to procedure.

- Keeping the skin taut to ensure maximum client comfort.

- Using correct soothing products to ensure maximum client comfort.

- Removing hair in direction of hair growth.

Eyebrow tinting-

- Cleansing and preparing eyebrow area prior to procedure.

- Protecting the skin around the area of which will be treated.

- Minimising the spread of colour to the surrounding environment, including clients clothes.

- Ensuring the product is applied neatly and evenly.

Artificial Eyelashes-

- Cleansing and preparing lashes prior to procedure.

- Ensuring the artificial lashes are positioned in an area that leaves the eye free of potential discomfort.

- Ensuring, upon application, that the artificial lashes are suitable for the discussed look and correctly positioned/merged with the natural eyelashes.

After treatment:

- Ensuring client is happy with initial results and has been fully informed of any aftercare procedures.

- Ensuring work station is left in a suitable condition for later treatment.

Waxing

In this module you would be expected to demonstrate an ability to perform waxing procedures, on areas such as the eyebrows, face, legs, underarms and bikini line. You must be able to identify the correct procedure for the correct client, help them prepare and plan for the treatment, and provide suitable aftercare advice. This module focuses heavily upon health, safety and hygiene standards.

As this is a module where you would be required to perform treatment, we have broken down some of the expected requirements needed to pass this module, into 'Before', 'During' and 'After' treatment.

Before treatment:

- Ensuring all tools and equipment are clean, using the correct methods.

- Ensuring client is in a comfortable position, to minimise pain, fatigue and possible cross infection during treatment.

- Ensuring the correct pre-wax products are used prior to waxing.

During treatment:

- Establishing hair growth pattern.

- Applying product according to the requirements of the hair growth pattern, and hair removal pattern.

- Ensuring client is comfortable throughout the waxing procedure.

- Minimising wastage of product during treatment.

After treatment:

- Ensuring that the client's treatment area is free of product and excess hair.

- Ensuring that the client has the correct aftercare advice, and is treated with correct soothing product.

Manicure

In this module, you would be expected to demonstrate an ability to perform manicure procedures, such as filing and buffing nails, massaging the hands and arms, providing suitable nail finishes and cuticle treatments. You must be able to identify the correct procedure for the correct client, help them prepare and plan for the treatment, and provide suitable aftercare advice. This module focuses heavily upon health, safety and hygiene standards.

As this is a module where you would be required to perform treatment, we have broken down some of the expected requirements needed to pass this module, into 'Before', 'During' and 'After' treatment.

Before treatment:

- Checking the desired shape and nail length with the client.

- Ensuring all tools and equipment are clean to industry standards.

- Removing all existing nail polish or product to ensure nails are treated while in natural condition.

- Disinfecting both your own, and client's hands.

During treatment:

- Filing the nails, to ensure smooth edges and desired shape.

- Using correct cuticle tools, to ensure minimised damage to both cuticle and nail plate.

- Utilising massage techniques to relax client.

- Using nail treatment to enhance the appearance of client's nails.

- Applying polish and top coats for desired finish.

After treatment:

- Ensuring nail plate is free of excess product, clean and dehydrated.

- Ensuring nail is left with a smooth texture, and the cuticle is free of debris.

- Ensure client has the correct aftercare advice.

Pedicure

In this module you would be expected to demonstrate an ability to perform pedicure procedures, such as nail filing, drying and cleansing feet, removing excess skin and performing foot and leg massage. You must be able to identify the correct procedure for the correct client, help them prepare and plan for the treatment, and provide suitable aftercare advice. This module focuses heavily upon health, safety and hygiene standards.

As this is a module where you would be required to perform treatment, we have broken down some of the expected requirements needed to pass this module, into 'Before', 'During' and 'After' treatment.

Before treatment:

- Disinfecting client's feet, to ensure treatment is performed under natural conditions.

- Identifying correct treatment, according to client's nail and skin condition.

- Consulting with client to identify desired nail length and finish.

During treatment:

- Cleaning and drying client's feet.

- Ensuring nails are filed, smoothed and shaped according to clients expectations.

- Removing any excess skin using correct tools and methods.

- Using correct massage techniques to ensure client relaxation.

After treatment:

- Ensuring that cuticle and nail plate are smooth and undamaged.

- Ensuring nails are left free of any debris or excess product.

- Ensuring client has correct aftercare advice.

Once you have completed Level 2, selected students will be invited to a Level 3 assessment day. This will involve a morning taster session, of both treatment and theory, and in the afternoon you will be required to complete a progression test. The type of test or question you will be asked, depends on the college you attend. This test is decided internally, but may include advanced theories such as:

- The endocrine system.

- Monitoring and application of spa treatment.

- Setting up and running promotional days and activities.

If you are successful in this endeavour, you will pass on to Level 3. Below we have listed some of the modules you might expect to encounter, if you progress.

Level 3 Modules

In these modules you should expect to encounter more advanced techniques than in the previous. You will be expected to demonstrate and take on more responsibility, learn and adapt to advanced treatments and display a higher level of customer care and initiative. These modules will vary from college to college.

Safety Monitoring

While Level 2 requires you to display a good understanding of the health and safety procedures within a salon, this module puts you in a senior position. Here, you are responsible for the monitoring of all persons upon the salon premises, and must ensure that all safety, statutory and work place instructions are carried out effectively and safely.

In this module you will be expected to demonstrate an understanding of:

- Health and safety regulations and workplace instructions.

- Monitory services, including monitory checks of the workplace at various times during the day to ensure a clean and safe environment.

- Ensure that salon workers are trained in health and safety and are able to apply this to their work.

Promotion and Sales

While Level 2 requires you to display a good understanding of how to promote and sell products to clients, in Level 3 you must demonstrate a further ability to plan, implement and evaluate possible promotional activities. You must also display the capability to work with others, to improve their promotional skills.

In this module you will be expected to demonstrate an understanding of:

- Recommending suitable promotional activities.

- Setting up and identifying realistic targets for proposed promotional activity.

- Ensuring promotional activity is fully planned and organised.

- Adapting promotional activity in response to issues or problems.

Body Massage Treatment

In this module you would be expected to demonstrate an ability to perform advanced massage treatments, such as massage of the head and body, and adapt and learn different massage techniques. The ability to identify the correct procedure for the correct client is more crucial in this module, and you must also be able to help the client prepare and plan for the treatment, and provide suitable aftercare advice. This module focuses heavily upon health, safety and hygiene standards.

As this is a module where you would be required to perform treatment, we have broken down some of the expected requirements needed to pass this module, into 'Before', 'During' and 'After' treatment.

d be required to perform treat-
e of the expected requirements
b 'Before', 'During' and 'After'

isinfected, post the prior treatment

stored according to manufacturing
vely energised.

ds the treatment procedure before it
with the sensation that will be created

o see how the client responds to both
es.

s supported and comfortable at all times

is protected against temperature during

ones are placed on the Chakra points, at the
eatment criteria.

llow smooth and easy movement of stones
g.

d disturbance is kept to a minimum durin

t during re-positioning process.

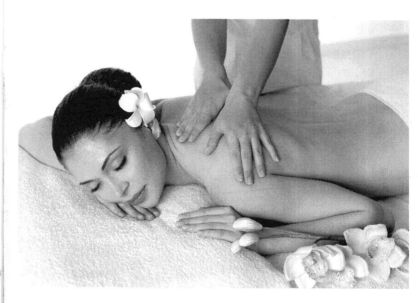

Before treatment:

- Consulting with client to explain and agree projected cost of treatment and frequency of potential further treatments.

- Consulting with client to identify medical history, lifestyle and any physical issues that may affect the treatment.

- Identifying correct treatment based on client's current physical condition.

- Preparing client's skin for the type of massage that will be performed.

- Ensuring client is correctly supported and comfortable prior to treatment.

- If using mechanical massage methods, ensuring client understands the sensation that they will experience.

- If using mechanical massage methods, ensuring that the correct treatment settings are used at all times.

During treatment:

- Adapting massage techniques according to treatment a client's physical requirement.

- Varying the depth and pressure of massage techniqu meet treatment objective, client's physical requirement preference.

- Utilising the correct application of massage oil.

- Ensuring client is comfortable at all times during the procedure

- Taking swift medical action if any discomfort occurs during the treatment.

After treatment:

- Allowing the client the correct post-treatment recovery period.

- Ensuring client is satisfied with finished result.

- Providing client with correct and sufficient aftercare advice.

Indian Head Massage

In this module you would be expected to demonstrate an ability to perform Indian head massage treatment, both with and without oils. The ability to identify the correct procedure for the correct client is more crucial in this module, and you must also be able to help the client prepare and plan for the treatment, and provide suitable aftercare advice. This module focuses heavily upon health, safety and hygiene standards.

As this is a module where you would be required to perform treatment, we have broken down some of the expected requirements needed to pass this module, into 'Before', 'During' and 'After' treatment.

As this is a module where you wou
ment, we have broken down some
needed to pass this module, int
treatment.

Before treatment:

- Ensuring stones have been c and pre the current.

- Ensuring stones have been instructions, and are effecti

- Ensuring client understand takes place, and is familiar by the stones.

- Carrying out a skin test t hot and cold temperature

Aft

- I(
  ti

- En:

- Ensu

Stone Th

In this modu
to perform h
massage and
to identify the c
in this module, a
plan for the trea
module focuses h

During treatment:

- Ensuring client's body during the procedure.

- Ensuring client's skin stone replacement.

- Ensuring the right std right times, to fulfil tr

- Lubricating skin to a to avoid overheatin

- Ensuring noise ar treatment.

- Assisting the clier

After treatment:

- Identifying and allowing the client allocated post-treatment recovery period.

- Ensuring the client is satisfied and happy with treatment results.

- Ensuring the client has the safe and correct aftercare advice.

As you can see from the above information, there are a wide range of abilities and skills you will need to display, in both Level 2 and Level 3. However, you should now have a good understanding of the type of practical exercise to expect. We will now move onto the exam section of the course, and the type of questions you should expect to encounter.

Sample Exam Questions

As we have already explained, a great deal of the learning during these modules will be science and anatomically based. This will be reflected in the exam papers you will take at the end of the year. You will need to undertake large amounts of revision for these papers, in order to memorise all of the information. These papers will involve a number of different types of question, ranging from True/False questions, to list questions and diagrams. To help you prepare for these examinations, we have helpfully included three tests containing 8 questions, highlighting the type of knowledge and skill you will be expected to produce. The following tests are based at Level 2. If you progress to Level 3, you should expect to see more advanced questions, covering topics such as the endocrine system.

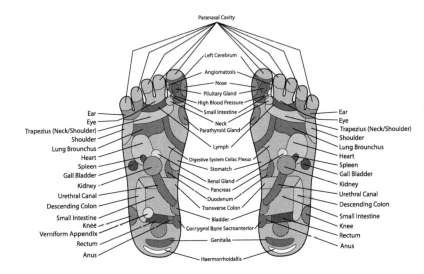

Test 1

Please answer the following questions with 'True' or 'False':

1. Paronychia is a bacterial infection. True or False?

2. If a client had mild dermatitis, you cannot provide any treatment in or around the nail area. True or False?

3. Potassium Hydroxide is present in cuticle remover. True or False?

4. An emollient is a cream based product. True or False?

5. Hand cream will only soften the skin and not the cuticles. True or False?

6. An oil manicure softens the cuticles. True or False?

7. Pterygium is the medical name for overgrown cuticles. True or False?

8. Paraffin wax treatment will cause sweating, allowing for a deeper cleanse. True or False?

Answers:

1. *True. Paronychia is a bacterial infection where the skin and nail meet at the base of a finger or toenail.*

2. *False. If a client has mild dermatitis, you can still provide a mild treatment to the surrounding/unaffected nail area.*

3. *True. Potassium Hydroxide is present in cuticle remover.*

4. *True. An emollient is a skin based product.*

5. *False. Hand cream will soften both the skin and cuticles.*

6. *True. An oil manicure softens the cuticles.*

7. *False. Pterygium is a growth that grows across the cornea of the eye.*

8. *True. Paraffin wax treatment will allow for a deeper cleanse.*

Test 2

1. What is the function of the nail plate?

2. What is the function of the nail matrix?

3. List 3 changes that can affect the nail as a result of ageing.

4. How many carpal bones are there in one hand and where would you locate them?

5. How many bones are there in each foot?

6. What is the name of the upper leg bone that extends from the pelvis to the knee?

7. What is the function of the cuticle?

8. Name the two bones in the lower leg.

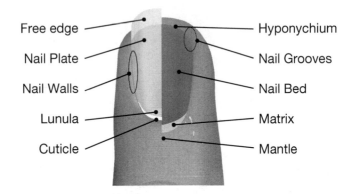

Free edge — Hyponychium
Nail Plate — Nail Grooves
Nail Walls — Nail Bed
Lunula — Matrix
Cuticle — Mantle

Answers:

1. The nail plate acts as a shield for the tissue underneath the nail bed.

2. The nail matrix is responsible for the production of cells which produce, and help to re-grow, the nail plate itself.

3. 3 changes that can affect the nails as a result of ageing are: Nails may become dull and brittle, tips may begin to fragment, and nails will grow more slowly.

4. There are 8 carpal bones in each hand, and they can be found on the wrist.

5. There are 26 bones in the human foot.

6. The name of the leg bone that extends from the pelvis to the knee is the femur.

7. The cuticle is a thin layer of skin that covers the nail plate and the nail root, just before the nail surfaces. It brings the skin and the nail plate together to provide a waterproof barrier.

8. The two bones in the lower leg are the Fibula and the Tibia.

Test 3

1. Name the 5 layers of the epidermis, starting from the inside to out.

2. List 10 bones of the face and cranium.

3. List 5 components of blood.

4. Give 3 functions of blood.

5. Where would you locate the Zygomaticus muscle?

6. Where would you locate the Trapezius muscle?

7. What is the largest muscle in the shoulder?

8. Where would you locate the Frontalis muscle, and what is its function?

Answers:

1. Stratum Basale, Stratum Spinosum, Stratum Granulosum, Stratum Lucidum, Stratum Corneum.

2. Frontal Bone, Nasal Bone, Parietal Bone, Temporal Bone, Lacrimal Bone, Zygomatic Bone, Ethmoid Bone, Sphenoid Bone, Vomer Bone, Mandible.

3. 5 components present in blood are: Plasma, Red Blood Cells, White Blood Cells, Platelets and Immunoglobulins.

4. 3 functions of blood are: To supply nutrients to the body, to remove waste from the body and to circulate white blood cells.

5. The Zygomaticus muscle is located in the cheek.

6. The Trapezius muscle is located between the neck and shoulders.

7. The largest muscle in the shoulder is the Deltoid Muscle.

8. The Frontalis muscle is located at the front of the head, it is used to lift the eyebrows.

How to become a Beauty Therapist

Hopefully, you should now have some idea of what to expect from a college course in beauty. Once you have completed your Level 3 examinations, or salon apprenticeship, you are ready to work within the industry. As a qualified beautician, there are several different options available. Later in the book, we will look at the different routes you might decide to take after completing your training, and help you reach a decision as to which one is right for you. In the next chapter, we will look at the other option available to aspiring therapists, in salon apprenticeships.

56

CHAPTER 5

Apprenticeship

After completing your GCSE's, you may you no longer wish to remain in the educatory system. This would rule out studying at college. Therefore, you might decide to apply for a salon apprenticeship. This involves going straight from school, into the workplace, and learning on-the-job. By the end of this process, you will have achieved exactly the same results as you would have from a standard college course, but on top of this you will also have valuable workplace experience. Some salons will have a training scheme, whereby a member of staff will spend 1 day a week of your apprenticeship, teaching you the same anatomical material as you would learn in college. Others may require you to spend 1 day a week in college, and the rest of the time performing practical theory as a junior member of staff. At the end of your apprenticeship, you will sit a very similar examination/ series of tests to those we listed in the previous chapter.

Many salons work directly as partners to local schools or colleges, in order to make this transition as smooth as possible. Salons generally look for candidates between the ages of 16-19, with C grades in both Maths and English. If the candidates do not have these grades, they will be required to take part in a separate course alongside their training, to get them to the required level.

There are both advantages, and disadvantages, to choosing this route instead of enrolling in a college course.

Advantages

- Your learning group will be much smaller than at college, which means you will have more one-to-one time with whomever is teaching you.

- You will earn money, while you learn.

- You will gain crucial industry experience from the frontline of a beauty salon.

- You will increase your employability, both by working with a potential future employer of the salon you are training in; and if you do have ambitions to work independently, will gain contacts and potential clients.

We asked our salon expert, who regularly takes on apprentices at her salon, what she feels the biggest advantage is:

'I feel that the apprenticeship option makes for a more confident therapist, both socially and professionally. College leavers are very nervous, very slow at treatments and often need training before they can work on clients. I have also found that therapists who took the apprentice option are far more comfortable in retailing products, and don't feel as if they are pressurising the client to buy.'

Disadvantages

- Working straight after leaving school leaves no time for 'growing up'.

- Often a small group dynamic can cause social issues.

Our resident expert elaborated on what she thinks is the biggest disadvantage of taking on apprentices:

'I believe the only disadvantage is that after a few months they can be overconfident. You sometimes have to pull them back, as they think they can do more than they are capable of. If they make a mistake, then the salon has to fix it.'

Application

In order to apply for a salon apprenticeship, candidates are required to send in a CV. The salon will then contact and invite the candidates to an interview. If you are someone who has recently finished their GCSEs, this can be an incredibly daunting process. However, it is important to remember that the interviewer themselves will recognise this, and will go easier on you as a result. The first step is to draft up a CV. If you are a younger candidate, you may not have any relevant work experience or training to fall back on. This is okay, since salons will expect this, and are looking for applicants who are eager to learn and develop.

In the next section we will draft a mock CV, which you can use as a basis for your own. We will later develop this CV, when showing you how to apply for salon work and jobs. As with any job application, you should start by writing a cover letter. A cover letter serves as a written introduction to your resume, and helps the employer get to know the candidate on a more personal level. In your cover letter you should include your skills and interests, why you are applying for the role, why you have chosen this particular apprenticeship/not to take a college course, and your future ambitions. If you have any past work related experience, this is also a great thing to include.

Cover Letter

Dear Sir/Madam,

I am writing to apply for a role as an apprentice at your salon. I feel this would be an ideal position for me. I recently completed my GCSE examinations and am really interested in going into the beauty industry. I have previous work experience as a receptionist in a local salon, and therefore already possess an understanding of what working in a salon will entail. I'm a really friendly, social person who loves to help people feel great about themselves, both in mind and body, and this is a role that would satisfy that. As an aspiring therapist, I would really love the opportunity to learn from established professionals such as yourself. Taking a salon apprenticeship would really enhance my future employability, not just within the beauty industry but within other customer service related fields too. It is my future aim to work within a salon, and this would provide invaluable experience for me. I'm an extremely hard worker, who loves to get hands on and learn new skills, and that is why I believe taking an apprenticeship is the best option. I'm the perfect person to learn on-the-job, and would make an enthusiastic addition to your group. I'd be very grateful if you could consider me for this position.

Yours sincerely,

Now that the reader has been introduced to you as a person, let's move onto your CV.

If you are someone aged 16, you may have limited experience with writing up CV's, or there is a good chance you may not have one at all. Here at How2Become, we will provide you with the best starting advice to help you through this process, and hopefully gain you an apprenticeship interview.

To start with, you need a good presentation, style or format to your document. A resume that is visually pleasing, and easy for an employer to gain information from, will instantly make a good impression. An employer must be able to find the qualities that they are looking for in your CV, within 11 seconds. Use the Cover Letter as a personal introduction, and then use your CV to present facts and information in an efficient manner. Your CV should contain:

- A brief personal profile
- Academic experience
- Employment history
- Work experience
- Key competencies and skills
- Hobbies and interests
- References

You should tailor these sections to meet the requirements of the position. For example, whilst 'having a friendly and sociable personality' wouldn't be particularly relevant if you were applying for a position as an IT Engineer, it is a vital part of working as a therapist, and therefore you should give this more credence in your skills list.

Below we have drafted up a sample CV that meets all of the necessary criteria, in both format and content. Write up your own, and see how it compares with ours.

For the purposes of this exercise, we have used fictitious personal details in reference to the example.

Example CV

Melanie Harris

Smith Street

Smith Town

Smithshire

Tel: 01634 123456

Email: MelanieHarris@emailaddresshere.com

Personal profile:

I am a well presented, articulate and aspiring beauty therapist, who has just completed her GCSE examinations. I'm very social and outgoing, I love to meet and help new people, and learn new skills in the process. I'm also a fantastic communicator, someone that people feel they can talk and relate with, and have great leadership skills. I have worked for one week as a receptionist in a salon in the past, and I have captained the girls hockey team at my previous school. I also acted as vice-captain for the football team. As a result, I already have a great understanding of what it means to work within a team, and how to be a great team member.

I've always been interested in beauty therapy, and frequently help my younger sister and my friends with their hair, makeup and nails. I consider no job too big, and would love to take on this challenge.

Academic experience:

Smith School for Girls:
GCSE Maths: C
GCSE English: C
GCSE History: B
GCSE French: D

Previous employment history:

Work experience at Smith's Street Spa, one week. Duties included: Cleaning, working reception, answering phone, making tea for customers.

Skills acquired from studying and work experience:

- GCSEs in Maths and English provide me with good communication, and numerical skills, which are useful for working at a reception.

- Work experience taught me the value of communicating effectively with customers, and keeping the salon clean and tidy.

- Science GCSE means that I already have some understanding of the human body, bone structure and anatomy.

- Experience of working as a team member, co-ordinating actions with other individuals in team and helping them, and consequently the team, to achieve higher goals.

Key competencies:

- Fantastic communicational and social skills.
- Great team working and leadership skills.
- Good numerical skills.
- Huge enthusiasm and interest for the beauty industry.

Significant achievements:

- Post and contribute regularly to various hair and beauty forums.
- Achieved a C in GCSE Maths and English.
- Completed a week of work experience at Smith's Street Spa.
- Led Hockey and Football teams to victory at school level.
- Regularly help friends and family with beauty tips and tricks.

Hobbies and interests:

When I am not working, I spend most of my time socialising with both my friends and family. I love to keep fit, and was a member of various sports teams at both school, and college level. I regularly post on hair and beauty forums, to ensure that I stay up to date with the latest trends and treatments available. I am someone who takes great value in my own appearance, and would love to instil this attitude on others.

References:

Available on request

As you can see from the way we have laid out our sample resume, it is important to ensure the employer can gain as much of the information they need, in as little time as possible. Just from a quick glance at our CV, you can immediately see that:

- We have GCSEs in Maths, English, History and Science.
- We completed 1 week of work experience at a beauty salon in the past.
- We have great teamwork and leadership skills.
- We are a social, articulate and relatable person, who would provide a friendly service to customers.

These are all key elements to working within a salon, and the fact that the reader can glean this information so quickly and easily, only makes the application more attractive. Particularly if you are someone without relevant work experience or employment history, it is even more important to display your strength of personality and personal achievements in the application.

Interview

If your application is successful, you will be invited to an interview with the salon. For apprenticeships, this will take the form of an informal chat, where the salon owner gets to know you and decides whether you are a suitable candidate as an apprentice. If are a younger candidate, you may not have any relevant experience with interviews. The process may be unfamiliar, and extremely daunting. Here at How2Become, we will provide you with the best advice possible for relaxing yourself prior to this interview, and passing the interview itself.

If you are not familiar with the process, here is how an interview works:

- The establishment will contact you via phone or email, to arrange a date and time in which you can come in and speak to them.

- When you arrive at the building, you will be invited into a room, either by a receptionist or the interviewer themselves. There is chance, for some jobs, that you may be interviewed by up to 3 different people. You will then sit down and begin the interview.

- The interview will last for around 20 to 30 minutes. This will consist of the person/persons asking you questions about yourself, your interest in working for the establishment, your future goals and ambitions and your knowledge of the selected field. You will then be invited to ask questions yourself.

- After leaving, you will be contacted after a short period of time, to let you know whether you were successful or not. The length of this period will vary from company to company.

In the next chapter of this book, we have listed a large number of potential interview questions, which you might expect to see if you were applying for an actual job in a salon. Since in this case, you are applying for an apprenticeship, the questions will be similar, but there will likely be less of them, and the interview itself will be less formal. The questions are also far more likely to be based around your personality, interest in the industry and work ethic, rather than requiring an in depth knowledge of the field. The salon knows that you are a beginner, and the interview will reflect this. That being said, we have still provided you with a number of questions that are unique and specific to working as an apprentice in a salon, and some sample answers on which you can base your own responses. This will help you prepare, and relax, for the interview ahead.

We asked our resident expert, who trains apprentices in her salon, what she thinks makes a good and bad candidate.

'A good candidate is someone who is on time, well spoken, meets the educational entry requirements, maintains good eye contact during the interview and is well presented. I look for candidates who maintain obvious care of their nails, wear light day make-up and have good personal hygiene. I also love candidates who ask questions, as this shows an interest in both me and my business.

A bad candidate, on the other hand, will have poor time keeping, appearance and communicational skills. Chipped nail polish is a big sign of this. I don't mind candidates who are shy, but if they can't hold a conversation with me then they won't be able to hold a conversation with clients, and that's fundamental to working in the industry.'

This statement should give you a great idea of what you should, and shouldn't do, during an interview. But what about what you should, and shouldn't say? Here at How2Become, we will guide you through the interview process. Using our expert's response, and our sample answers, you should have no problem passing an interview for a salon apprenticeship.

1. Why are you interested in doing an apprenticeship, instead of going to college?

This is a question you should expect to see in almost every apprenticeship interview you attend. The interviewer is asking for confirmation of the fact that you understand, on a basic level at the very least, the differences between working as an apprentice and taking a college course. The interviewer is also asking you to elaborate on what you feel the benefits of working as an apprentice are, and how this is more suitable for you personally as opposed to going to college. At the start of the chapter we provided you with a range of different advantages that working as an apprentice can bring. Use these to construct your answer.

Write your answer in the box provided, and then compare it with the sample response below.

Sample response:

I'm interested in doing an apprenticeship for a number of reasons. Firstly, I'm someone with a hard work ethic, who is really interested in working within the beauty industry. I feel that learning on the job would be much more beneficial and interesting than attending college. I want to be on the frontline so to speak, and the opportunity to learn directly from professionals such as yourself would be hugely advantageous to my future career prospects. I'd like to work in a salon full time, and the experience this could provide me surpasses anything I believe I could learn within college. I'm really keen to further my employability skills, and I think this is the best way to do it.

2. Why do you want to work as an apprentice for this salon?

This is another, very popular question. Just as they would in a regular job interview, the salon is looking for some confirmation of the fact you have researched them beforehand, and that they have qualities that are attractive to you. Don't be afraid to flatter the salon here. Use the internet to research particular products, services and treatments that the salon offers, which you can then mention in the interview; ring the salon prior to the interview and enquire as to what services they offer (if they don't have a website) or even go in and have a treatment. Mention the atmosphere of the salon and the friendliness of the staff as positive reasons for your decision to apply.

Write your answer in the box provided, and then compare it with the sample response below.

Sample response:

Well, there are a number of different things that attracted me to this salon. Aside from the location, as it's just five minutes away, I know you perform Rose Body and Facial treatments. From doing internet research, and hearing friends and family talk about these treatments, I'm really interested to give them a go. I'm also excited about the idea of performing Electrolysis and Reflexology, both of which I know are offered here at this salon. I've been into this salon before, and the staff were always so friendly and helpful; I'd love to be a part of that atmosphere, and hopefully I could bring some new ideas and lots of enthusiasm to the team. My Mum and I are huge users of their products, so it would be great to promote and sell these in the future.

3. What makes you a unique candidate?

This question is essentially asking you to sell yourself, as you would a product in the salon. The asker wants to know the reasons why they should consider you, over other applicants. It is a great question, as it allows you to talk about your strengths as a candidate and why the salon should take you on as an apprentice. Take a deep breath before answering, think about your response and structure it so that the salon understands exactly why you would make an ideal candidate for the apprenticeship. Remember all the positive qualities we listed in the CV, and consider exactly how these can be applied to a role in a beauty salon.

Write your answer in the box provided, and then compare it with the sample response below.

Sample response:

There are many different qualities that set me apart from other candidates. First of all, I believe my enthusiasm for the role is unmatched. I'm hugely interested in the beauty industry, I subscribe regularly to beauty forums, magazines and websites, and I'm absolutely meticulous when it comes to my appearance. I'd love to use these values within the professional environment, and I think I'd be a great representative for your salon in this respect. Secondly, my teamwork and leadership skills are at an extremely high level. As a competitive sports woman at school, and captain of both hockey and football, I have a fantastic understanding of the unity and co-operation required to work within, and lead a team, and I would use these skills within the workplace. Lastly, my work experience at Smith Street Salon gives me vital previous experience and knowledge of the work place environment. I can put the skills I picked up from this role to immediate and effective use. I'm someone who really wants to improve, better myself and learn new skills, and this salon would be the perfect place for me to do that.

The following chapter will cover more potential questions, which you might expect see when applying for either a job, or apprenticeship at a salon. Let's move onto the next stage of the interview.

Asking Questions

Before you leave the salon, the interviewer will ask, 'Do you have any questions?' This is a hugely important part of the interview process, and one where many candidates fall down. You should always aim to show the salon that you are interested and enthusiastic in working for them, and therefore the worst thing you can say here is 'I don't know'. Prior to the interview, prepare a list of 7 to 8 questions that you can ask in this situation. That way, even if one, two or three of your questions are covered by the information given to you during the interview, you will still be prepared with more. Questions can include the following:

- What training will I receive, and how will the learning process compare to college?
- How many non-practical hours of work per week are there?
- Do you offer a personal training programme, or do candidates also need to register for college?
- What wage do you pay your apprentices?
- If I was successful in my application, what would you expect from me? How fast would you expect me to develop my skills?
- Is there a potential job opportunity at the end of the apprenticeship?
- When do the final assessments/ non practical exams take place?

If you are successful in your application, you will begin training immediately with the salon. Your weekly hours and activities would depend on the establishment in which you are working, and how the salon owner wishes to structure your learning. In the next chapter, we will provide you with more potential interview questions, should you apply to work full time within a salon after your apprenticeship. Following this, in chapter 7, we'll elaborate upon exactly what jobs you will be expected to perform when working full time in a salon, and how to manage your time. As a salon apprentice, you will spend much of your time assisting and learning from these employees in their everyday professional life, and therefore both of these chapters will be extremely useful to you.

CHAPTER 6

Salon Interview

In this chapter we will teach you the application and interview skills needed to gain employment in a salon. By the end of this chapter you will have a full working knowledge of the type of questions to expect if you attend a salon interview, and the best way to answer them.

As a salon worker, you will normally work from 9-5, up to 5 days a week. Clients will book specific treatments, and you will be expected to perform these treatments to high standards. Your work will normally begin and end 1 hour before the salon opens and closes for business, since there are large amounts of preparation to be done in both preparing the salon for the day ahead, and cleaning, ready for the next day.

Application

As with any job, the first step you should take is to look for vacancies. This can be done in a number of different ways. If there is a local salon in your vicinity, drop by and hand them your CV. This is a better approach than applying online, as most local salons are small, independently run businesses. Your resume is likely to go straight through to the manager, and there is even a good chance that you will be handing in your application to the manager themselves. This gives you a great opportunity to make an initial impression, and pre-sell yourself before they have read your application form. It is a good idea to send or hand in your CV at multiple salons, instead of focusing on just one in particular.

The other option involves downloading an online application form, and sending it in. If you are downloading the application form directly from the company website, you should expect to see something similar to this:

Name:

Age:

Address:

Email:

Nationality:

Title of post you are applying for:

The application form will then question your beauty experience. This is where you must sell yourself, pre-interview, to the salon. We have listed some of the questions you might expect to see in a salon application form, and how to answer them.

1. How would you deal with a client who was dissatisfied with the treatment or service that you provided?

This question is asking for a number of different things. Chiefly, it is looking for you to show initiative and responsibility in dealing with clients. It is also looking for you to highlight your communicational ability, to decide on the best possible resolution for the client. In order for a salon to hire you, they need to know they are taking on board someone who can be trusted to deal with clients in a calm and relaxed manner, not someone who will cause conflict for potential returnees.

Write out your answer in the box provided, and then see how it compares with the sample response below.

Sample Response:

In the unlikely event that a client was unhappy with the service I provided, I would calmly and clearly enquire as what they are unhappy with, apologise sincerely and then endeavour to fix the issue to the best of my ability. If I had another client waiting, I would make sure they are comfortable and aware of the time frame in which they should expect to wait, before ensuring my current client leaves as happy as possible. If, after attempts to fix the treatment they are still not satisfied, (upon discussion with the manager) I would offer them a refund or free future treatment.

2. What would you do if a client had a bad reaction to the products you were using?

This question is looking for you to demonstrate your knowledge of health and safety, and contra-indication procedure. Instead of giving a general answer here, you can utilise the skills you have learned and give some different examples of safety procedure, upon unexpected or allergic client reaction to a product. Use this question to display both your customer service skills, and your safe and reliable persona.

Write out your answer in the box provided, and then see how it compares with the sample response below.

Sample Response:

If a client had a bad reaction to the products I was using, then the first thing I would do, would be to immediately stop the treatment. I would enquire with the customer as to exactly what sensation they are feeling, and where they are feeling it. I would then apply the necessary health and safety steps. This would depend on the issue, or treatment type, but some examples might be:

Burning or stinging during eye treatment: Making sure the clients clothes are protected, and their eyes are closed, use a bowl of warm water and clean cotton wool to bathe the eyes. I would run the water from the tear duct to the corner of the eye, before letting the water drizzle back into the bowl. I would repeat this process until the pain has subsided, and apologise to the client.

Burning during a wax treatment/wax too hot: I would immediately stop the treatment and apply a soothing/cooling product to the skin, as well as letting the prepared wax cool down slightly, in order to prevent further issues. I would then apologise to the client.

3. What would you do if you were running late for a treatment?

Similarly to the first question, this is asking you to display your initiative. A short and simple answer here will suffice, just ensure that you display both your impeccable customer service, and organisational skills.

Write out your answer in the box provided, and then see how it compares with the sample response below.

Sample response:

If I was running late for a treatment then I would endeavour to let the client whose treatment has been delayed, know as soon as possible. I would try to give the client as accurate an estimation as possible of when I will be able to perform the treatment, and if this does not suit their needs, try to arrange a later appointment for when I am free. This may be during my scheduled lunch break. If the client does decide to wait, I would try to ensure they are as comfortable as possible whilst waiting.

4. What are your strengths as a beauty therapist?

As a reader of this guide, this is a perfect question. We have already highlighted on several occasions just what strengths you need to succeed within the beauty industry, and therefore you should have a great idea of how to answer this question. Make sure you draw attention to your social skills, love of meeting new people, customer handling and interest in beauty.

Write out your answer in the box provided, and then see how it compares with the sample response below.

Sample response:

My biggest strength as a beauty therapist is my bubbly and social personality. I love meeting, talking to and finding out new things about people, and that is why I would be perfect for this job. I trained at college and have a Level 3 Diploma, so I am fully experienced with the procedures and treatments that I would be required to perform while working at this salon. I've always been good at helping people, both on a personal and physical level, and this is a job that would combine both of those skills. I am particularly interested in the changing nature of the beauty industry, and excited to adapt my methods to include new and modern treatments, year on year.

5. What are your weaknesses as a beauty therapist?

This is an interesting question, and one you should answer carefully, but honestly. Don't reel off a list of weaknesses, but focus more on one particular quality that you would like to improve, and how working in a beauty salon can help you to improve that attribute. This will show the salon that you are both honest, and willing to learn.

Write out your answer in the box provided, and then see how it compares with the sample response below.

Sample response:

My biggest weakness as a beauty therapist is in my organisational ability. While I fully understand the need for good time management as a therapist, I have not always been so capable of applying this in the past. However, I fully believe that working in a salon will give me the experience required to solve this issue, and that it is something that can easily be overcome. I am eager to improve and learn in every area, not just organisationally but as a person overall, and I believe working in a salon can really enhance my abilities.

6. What are your career goals?

This is another area we have already touched on. In answering this question you should show an enthusiastic approach, which demonstrates that you are ambitious, and that you have thought about how the salon will help you grow as a beauty therapist. Don't be scared to tell the salon that you would like to open your own salon someday, or teach beauty. They are looking for an applicant who is willing to learn, improve new skills and develop the capability to run the salon in the absence of senior management.

Write out your answer in the box provided, and then see how it compares with the sample response below.

Sample response:

In the future, I hope to open and run my own salon. However, I currently lack both the experience and management skills required to do this. I really believe that by working at this salon, I will develop the capabilities required to progress up to a high enough level to achieve this. I see this as an institution that I could work at long term, for several years, and perhaps one day progress to the level of senior management within the salon. I believe working here would be a fantastic opportunity for me, and that I could provide an excellent and refreshing service for both you and your clients.

7. What is it about this salon in particular that interests you, and why do you think you would make a good member of the team?

This is a question that requires you to demonstrate both a level of prior research, and team experience. The research should be simple enough. Go onto Google and search for the salon, if they have a website then they should also have a list of the type of treatments available. Take 3 of these treatments, and insert them into your answer, using them as a reason for why you are interested in working at this salon. Location and salon atmosphere may also be influences for why you have applied for the role. In terms of teamwork, if you lack any direct team experience then simply demonstrate that you are an outgoing, social and friendly person who is willing to work with anyone you meet.

Write out your answer in the box provided, and then see how it compares with the sample response below.

Sample response:

This salon really appealed to me, because of both the type of treatments it provides, and atmosphere when I have come in before. In terms of location, the salon is perfect for me to get to, and whenever I've had treatments here in the past all of the staff have been so warm, friendly and inviting. I feel that fits in perfectly with the service I can provide. I am really interested in Rose Facial Treatments, CACI detoxifying massages and working with high quality products. My diploma in Level 3 Beauty has also provided me with experience in other treatments that your salon currently runs, such as hot stone massages, and Indian head massages.

'While I do not have direct team experience, I am an optimistic, friendly person who takes great pleasure in working as a group member to produce effective results. I always get along with people

and would have no trouble in applying this attitude towards working at your salon. I believe that I would be a fantastic, reliable and hard-working addition to any salon team.'

'My experience working at my local fast food restaurant has taught me the value of teamwork, as I spent almost every day working there as a member of a team, both dealing with customers and cooking products. I learned the importance of time management, discipline, co-ordination and unity as a member of the restaurant team and I believe this is something that would aid me greatly whilst working in a salon.'

Following this, the application may then ask you for a list of the experience or training you undertook at both Level 2, and Level 3, as well as the necessary equal opportunities enquiries.

C.V.

If, in the event the salon does not have an application form, you will need to persuade them via your CV, and cover letter. These can be tricky, but luckily here at How2become, we have the knowledge and tools to help you through this process. In this section, we will craft both an ideal cover letter, and CV, to help you persuade beauty salons to invite you for an interview.

Let's start with the cover letter. A cover letter should serve as an introductory statement, prior to your CV. You need to keep the readers interest, but keep your opening statement short and sweet. Let them know who you are, what your interests are, why you are applying for the job and what you think you can bring to their beauty salon.

Write out your sample cover letter in the box provided, and then see how it compares with our cover letter below.

Dear Sir/Madam,

I am writing to apply for the role of junior beauty therapist. I feel that this would be a perfect position for me. I recently completed my Level 3 Diploma in Beauty Therapy, and am now looking to gain crucial experience within the industry. As someone who is friendly, sociable and loves to help people feel good about themselves, both mentally and physically, I am looking to further my industry skills by learning from established professionals within the field. I have always been interested in beauty, and this has only been enhanced by my college studies. I already possess excellent customer service skills and experience, through my time working at the restaurant, and via my college course I have gained a great deal of knowledge about many of the treatments you currently provide in your salon. I will bring a wealth of new ideas, and would be an enthusiastic, hard-working and reliable addition to your team. I really hope that you will consider me for this position.

Yours sincerely,

Now that we have the reader's attention, let's move onto the CV.

As with any job, you should tailor your CV to meet the requirements of the position. It is estimated that employers look at a CV for all of 11 seconds, and if they cannot find the information they require, discard the application. Therefore, we need to be succinct, clear and to the point with both our wording and presentation. The salon needs to know immediately that you are in possession of the qualities they are looking for.

Below we have drafted up an ideal CV that meets all of the necessary criteria, in both format and content. If you already have a CV, take it out and compare it with our draft. For the purposes of this exercise, we have used fictitious persona details in our example.

Beauty Therapist CV

Melanie Harris
Smith Street
Smith Town
Smithshire
Tel: 01634 123456
Email: MelanieHarris@emailaddresshere.com

Personal profile:

I am a well presented, articulate and capable junior beauty therapist, who has just completed her Level 3 Diploma in Beauty Therapy. My studies have taught me the skills to perform a variety of different treatments with the utmost confidence and care for the customer. I am a fantastic communicator who relates well with everybody I meet, and am able to work effectively as part of a team, and individually. I consider no job too big, and through both my experience working at a restaurant, and college, understand the requirements of working in a fast paced, customer service related environment.

Academic experience:

Smith school for girls:
GCSE Maths: C
GCSE English: C
GCSE History: B
GCSE French: D

Smith College:
NVQ Level 2 Beauty Therapy: Pass
NVQ Level 3 Beauty Therapy: Pass

Previous employment history:

Smith Restaurant, 2010-2012

Duties included cleaning, cooking, dealing face to face with customers, working extensively as part of a team and on night shifts, individually. Have managed backroom at times of understaffing and worked as senior till manager.

Skills acquired from studying and past employment:

- Extensive knowledge of past and current beauty treatments, including: Indian head massage, hot stone treatment, facial skin treatment, eyebrow waxing, pedicures and manicures.

- Learned how to communicate with customers and clients to provide a service that satisfies their needs and requirements.

- Detailed understanding of anatomy, bone structure and pressure points in the human body.

- Experience of working as a team member, co-ordinating actions with other individuals and helping them to achieve higher goals.

- Experience in promoting and selling products to clients.

Key competencies:

- Fantastic communicational and social skills.

- Strong experience in upselling and promoting products.

- Great understanding of health and safety procedures and customer care/satisfaction.

- Experience with a variety of different treatments, as well as keeping up to date with new treatments.

Significant achievements:

- Post and contribute regularly to various hair and beauty forums.

- Achieved a pass in both Level 2 and Level 3 Beauty at college.

- Successfully completed a three week course in first aid.

- Acted as a counselling representative for college whilst studying.

- Regularly help friends and family with beauty tips and tricks.

Hobbies and interests:

When I am not working, I spend most of my time socialising with both my friends and family. I love to keep fit, and was a member of various sports teams at both school, and college level. I regularly post on hair and beauty forums, to ensure that I stay up to date with the latest trends and treatments available. I am someone who takes great value in my own appearance, and would love to instil this attitude on others.

References:

Available on request

As you can see from our example, when writing a CV you should be direct and to the point. Just from a quick glance, looking at the layout of our draft, an employer would immediately be able to tell that:

- We have Diplomas at both Level 2 and Level 3 in Beauty Therapy.
- We have worked in the service industry and therefore have customer service experience.
- We have skills and interest in various different treatment procedures.
- We have good communicational ability.
- We have GCSEs in English and Maths.

These are all key elements to working within a beauty salon, and all of these have been shown without even reading the personal profile. Particularly in a big salon, employers will receive hundreds of these applications, and therefore it is a great idea to make your presence felt quickly and effectively. Do not waste their time with long paragraphs or statements, bullet points are a far more effective way to put across your skillset and experience.

Interview

If the salon likes what they have read, you will be invited to an interview. If you are unsure of the location of the salon, it is a good idea to practice different routes of getting there prior to the interview, to ensure you aren't late. In particular for a beauty interview, you should do your best to present yourself correctly, and dress smartly.

Salons are looking for employees who share the same values as they do, and who will present these values outwardly to the cliental.

Interviews can be an extremely nerve wracking process. While you may have had experience interviewing for college, actual employment can be an entirely different matter, and the interviewers themselves may have stricter requirements. Therefore it is a good idea, prior to your interview, to research both the salon, and the type of questions you might be asked. You can then practice these questions to yourself, friends or family, to prepare for the interview situation. You should also have a detailed and complete knowledge of your CV, since many employers will adapt their questions towards this.

Here at How2become, we have tracked down a number of different, beauty salon interview questions, and helpfully included them all below. By using this guide, you will have nothing to worry about when it comes to the actual interview. The less nervous you are, the more confident you will come across, and the better chance you will have of getting the job.

1. Tell me about yourself.

This is a common question, and one that is often used to relax the interviewee. As we have highlighted several times, personality is the single most important aspect for potential beauty therapists, and therefore the asker here is simply looking for you to put across your sociable, and friendly personality, in as clear and concise a manner as possible. They want to get to know you, in the same way your clients might, and therefore this is a great opening question.

Write your answer in the box provided, and then compare it with the sample answer below.

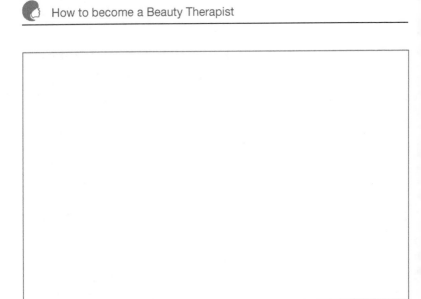

Sample response:

I'm a sociable and friendly person, who is really interested in the beauty industry. I love meeting and getting to know new people, which is one of the reasons I applied for this role. I also love counselling and helping others, and I think this job will allow me to do that, both on a physical and mental level. I've recently completed my Level 3 NVQ in beauty therapy at Smith College, and now I'm looking to work in an actual salon.

2. What are your strongest qualities?

Prior to your interview, make a list of your strongest qualities. Not only will this prepare you for the question, but it will work as a confidence building tool. Then take the most important qualities from that list, and order them in terms of importance to the role you are applying for. Find examples of when you have used these strong points, and structure them into a response which tells the employer why they should hire you.

Write your answer in the box provided, and then compare it to our sample answer below.

Sample response:

Well firstly, I'm extremely sociable. I know that it's important to have a friendly and relatable personality in this industry, and that is one of the reasons I believe I'm so suited to the role. While I was at college, I volunteered as a member of the college counselling team, offering personal advice to younger and more troubled students. I'm a great listener and it was highly rewarding to make a difference. I'm also really interested in the industry as a whole. I regularly post on hair and beauty forums, purchase magazines and keep up to date with the latest trends and treatments. I really enjoyed taking my Level 3 at college, because it gave me advanced, hands on experience with some of the treatments I had read about; I just love the way the beauty industry is always changing and there are always new things to learn. Working at a restaurant has taught me great customer service, and teamwork skills, so I'd like the chance to apply these to a job I'm interested in.

3. Why do you think you'd do well at this job?

While the previous question asked for a summary of your best skills, now you need to show how you would apply these skills to the role. Take each skill that you mentioned, and evaluate exactly how it would help you to succeed within this position.

Write your answer in the box provided, and then compare it with the sample answer below.

Sample response:

Well, as I said, I'm a very sociable person, and find it easy to relate with people, so I think I would have no problems building up a rapport with clients. I know that clients often just need someone who will listen to them, and I'm very happy to do that. I'm really excited to learn and improve my treatment technique too. Studying at college gives you lots of experience, but there is a ceiling; I really feel that working in a salon is the next stage for me. I can't think of anything better than making clients feel happy and good about themselves, inside and out. At my local restaurant I had lots of experience of dealing with unhappy customers whilst working on the till; and I think this will really help me; especially in the beauty industry where people are so particular and perfectionist about their looks. I value, and take great pride in my appearance, so I think I'd be a perfect representative for your salon.

4. What motivates you?

In this question, the interviewer is essentially asking you to show them why and how you would be a motivated, long term employee, who won't get bored with the role and leave within a few months. They are looking for someone who is interested and willing to learn new skills, who will take on challenges that might be considered more difficult for a junior beauty therapist.

Write your answer in the box provided, and then compare it with the sample response below.

Sample response:

I'm a very motivated person. Personally, I'm motivated by a desire to help people, and make them feel better about themselves. I'm also someone who is constantly trying to improve her own appearance, I'm very meticulous in that respect, and I'd love to help other people improve their own. Professionally, I'm motivated by the idea of learning and improving. I loved my Level 3 Beauty course, because it taught me so much about anatomy and different treatment types, but now I want the opportunity to put what I've learned into practice. I think working here could teach me so much more about the industry, and it's definitely somewhere I could see myself working for several years.

5. Why should we hire you, over other candidates?

When answering this question, take a deep breath beforehand. Many people hear this question and rush into a big, convoluted list that only tells the employer one thing, you are not right for the role. Consider the qualities you listed in the previous questions, and find a way to make these qualities sound unique, interesting and persuasive. Think about yourself as a product, why should the salon buy into you? A good way to prepare for this question is to write a list of all your qualities, and how you would bring them to the position. Make sure you draw attention to your professional ambitions, so the employer can see that you are someone who is dedicated to the cause.

Write your answer in the box provided, and then compare it with the sample response below.

Sample response:

Well, I believe that you should hire me for a number of reasons. Firstly, I feel it would be hard to match my enthusiasm for the role. I've been interested in beauty since I was a little girl, I learnt how to do my hair and makeup from my mother and I have passed those skills down to both my friends and my little sister. As I mentioned, I subscribe regularly to several beauty magazines, and am a consummate member of online websites and forums that detail the latest trends and advancements in the industry. My work counselling at college also gives me a huge edge. I know that clients need a good, sympathetic listener, and someone who can relate with them, and I firmly believe I am the right person to provide that service to your customers. The customer service and teamwork skills that I picked up from my time working in a restaurant will aid me greatly in this endeavour. As a Level 3 student, I already have advanced knowledge of many of the treatments that you offer in your salon and would come into the role fully prepared to perform to the best of my ability.

Overall, I just want to learn, improve and better myself. It is my ulti-mate goal to open my own salon, and I really believe this is the best place to prepare me for that.

6. What are your weaknesses?

Similarly to the application form answer, here you should focus on one particular weakness, and how much you would like to improve in this area. This will show the salon that you are honest about your own limitations, and that you are someone who is willing to learn and grow with the role. Keep it short, to the point and don't be scared to flatter the employer, by letting them know that you think they are the best person to help you improve.

Write your answer in the box provided, and then compare it with the sample response below.

Sample response:

I would say that my biggest weakness is in my organizational ability, and time management skills. I know that working in a salon is a role that demands good initiative in both of these categories, and therefore it is something I am really hoping to learn and improve upon whilst I work here. The chance to learn from professionals such as yourself will only aid me in this venture.

7. What is your aim for the future?

In this question you should show that you are an ambitious individual who is looking to progress to a higher level within the industry. There is nothing wrong with telling the salon that you have future ambitions to start your own business, or to teach beauty to younger students. They will appreciate that they are interviewing someone with the desire to learn, who will put their experience to good use. Just make sure that you tell the salon that you see yourself as working for them for a number of years. A salon is highly unlikely to employ you, for example, if you tell them that within the next year you are aiming to open your own salon and won't be staying in the role.

Write your answer in the box provided, and then compare it with the sample response below.

Sample response:

Well, in the immediate future I hope to be an employee of this salon. If I'm successful, I can easily see myself working here for a number of years, and hopefully will progress to the level where I can either train younger staff, or manage the salon in the absence of yourself. I'm a very ambitious person, so in the long term, it's my goal to set up my own salon. Obviously, that's a long way off, and I have many years of training to complete before I can even think of achieving it, but it's certainly something that I'm working towards for the future. If I can't achieve that, then I would love to teach beauty, either in a college or privately. I love helping people and as a long term ambition, that is something that is very achievable. I believe your salon is the best place for me to improve myself enough to accomplish these aims.

8. What do you know about our salon?

This question is looking for a demonstration of research, prior to the interview. Make sure you go into the salon beforehand, or Google search them, to gain all the possible information that you can. Take note of: what year they opened, changes in management, what the staff are wearing, what treatments they offer and any rare or special procedures they perform, the types of products they offer and the name of those products, what brands the salon works with and the atmosphere of the salon. All of these can be used in your answer. This question is where you can flatter the interviewer, and their salon, with enthusiasm towards working for their particular institution. Roughly speaking, this question translates as, 'Why do you want to work here, and not elsewhere?'

Write your answer in the box provided, and then compare it with the sample response below.

Sample response:

Well I've actually been a customer here on a number of occasions, and it was a fantastic experience. My therapist made me look and feel absolutely great, and that was one of the reasons I applied to work at this salon. Every time I come in for a treatment, the atmosphere is so warm and friendly and I'd love to be a part of that. I know you've been open since 2007, and that you yourself have been the manager since then. I also know that you offer unique treatments and products such as Rose Facials, which aren't available in every salon. I'm also really excited to work with Electrolysis, as this was something we covered on my college course, and I found extremely fascinating. In terms of location this salon is also perfect for me, it's five minutes from my house and that means I can be here early every single morning, to help prepare and set up for the day ahead.

9. Tell me about a time you have dealt with a difficult customer?

You should expect to see a couple of these questions, particularly when working in a customer service related field such as beauty. The salon needs to know that it is hiring someone who is capable of dealing with unhappy clients, and ensuring said clients will return for further treatment. When detailing the incident, make sure you don't just list the incident itself. Tell the interviewer how you dealt with the issue and ensured that the customer was satisfied and likely to return for further products. Make your answer as clear and concise as possible, so the interviewer sees exactly what the issue was, why it occurred and how you solved it.

Write your answer in the box provided, and then see how it compares with the sample response below.

Sample response:

When I worked at my local restaurant, this was a frequent issue. In particular since my restaurant was within a Motorway premises, we often had tired and unhappy customers stopping off to buy food. As a member of the till you are a frontline representative for the company and must behave accordingly. Whenever we had complaints they were dealt with swiftly and effectively. One such instance was when a customer returned their product, which had been contaminated pre-purchase, by factors in store. The customer was irate and demanding to speak to someone in senior management. As a customer service representative, I politely and fairly persuaded the individual to calm down, apologised sincerely, gave them a full replacement and issued some of their payment back. The customer left satisfied and happy with their meal, and that their issue had been fixed.

10. Tell me about a time you have used your initiative, to help your team?

Similarly to the last question, this is asking for direct examples of a time when you have demonstrated the sort of behaviour the salon would expect from you, whilst working for them. In your answer you should focus on the value of teamwork, your appreciation and understanding of team dynamics and how you helped your team to succeed.

Write your answer in the box provided, and then see how it compares with the same response below.

Tell me about a time you have used your initiative, to help your team?

Answer: As a crew member at my local restaurant, team work was integral to the role. I frequently worked in teams of 3 to 4 people, to ensure that product was made as efficiently and effectively as possible. This often involved working during rush hour shifts, where the atmosphere was fast paced and highly stressful. One incident I can remember was when, upon finishing my own product, I noticed that the team member next to me was struggling with his workload. Upon ensuring there were no immediate requirements on my part, I swiftly coordinated myself to help him get up to speed with his task; resulting in as little delay to the production as possible. I have also trained new team members, and led the backroom during busy periods.

11. Do you have any questions for me?

By the time this question is asked, you will have reached the end of the interview. This is an extremely important stage, as it is vital to leave the interviewer with a lasting, good impression. The absolute worst thing you can say here is 'no'. This shows a lack of interest, enthusiasm and passion for the role. Write down several questions prior to the interview, so that even if two or three of your answers are covered over the course of the questioning, you will still have questions left to ask at the end. Make sure when you ask these you are as enthusiastic as you have been throughout the rest of the interview. If you are really struggling for questions, find something that you already know the answer to (prior to the interview) and then ask anyway. Create a workflow chart, with expected answers, where you can ask a question, receive an answer, and then follow up with another question based on the previous answer you have received.

Write your questions in the box provided, and then see how they compare with ours. Try to come up with at least 7 different questions.

Do you have any questions for me?

How much does the job pay?

What are the hours like?

What kind of treatments would I start off performing?

Is there any training involved?

What are the company values?

How does the salon obtain details with the brands you promote?

Will there be an opportunity to visit roadshows or beauty markets?

What's the number one thing you look for in an employee of your salon?

Top interview tips

- **Research.** Prior to the interview, make sure you know details of when the salon was opened, the type of treatments offered, the type of products they sell and the type of values they promote.

- **Practice.** Practice as many questions and answers with friends or family as you possibly can. If you go through enough potential questions, there is no way you can be surprised by anything the interviewer asks. Confidence is key, and the more confidence you exude, the more likely you are to get the job.

- **Good eye contact.** When being interviewed, ensure you maintain good eye contact with the interviewer. Particularly in a beauty salon, where social skills are given high priority, you will need to show the interviewer that you are someone with great body language and communicational abilities.

- **Dress appropriately.** Similar to the last point, a beauty salon is an institution that promotes pride and care in personal appearance. Therefore they will be looking to employ someone who shares the same values.

- **Sell yourself.** Remember that you are there to promote yourself as an individual, much like you would a product to a customer. You need to show the interviewer exactly why you are the right person for the role

- **Breath.** This is a useful, and commonly used trick. Whenever you are asked a question, lean back, take a deep breath and think about your answer. The interviewer will not judge you for considering carefully what to say. Another common trick when faced with a question is to ask the interviewer to repeat the question, to give you more time to think of a suitable answer.

CHAPTER 7

Salon Worker

If you are successful with your interview, you will be offered a job at the salon. In this chapter, we will highlight exactly what you should expect from the role. We will explore the day to day duties that a salon or spa therapist must perform, and the challenges you might face. In this chapter, we have taken two real life experiences of salon therapists that we interviewed, and provided you with a daily time-line of their duties. We hope this gives you a better understanding of exactly what the role entails. Our two therapists are named Sandra and Julie. Let's meet them.

Sandra is a beauty therapist from Croydon. She works 9-5 in a small, local salon five days a week, including Saturdays. We have laid out her regular day, to give you a good idea of what to expect when working in a salon.

Julie is a beauty therapist from Ashford. She runs her own, local salon and works from 9-5 most days of the week. Julie performs both treatment, and management tasks, on a day to day basis. We have laid out her regular day, to give you a good idea what to expect when running your own salon.

Sandra

08:00

At 08:00, Sandra arrives at the salon. Her day actually begins at 09:00, but it is important that she arrives early, in order to help get the salon prepared and ready for the day's treatments. Her first treatment is a short, fifteen minute eyebrow wax. In order to prepare for the day, Sandra must perform activities such as:

- Heating towels
- Turning on the heating so the salon is warm for clients
- Lighting candles
- Making fresh coffee

- Checking the answer machine, and ringing people to confirm their appointments

As Sandra's first treatment is a waxing treatment, she must also turn on the wax in advance to make sure it is in the right condition to perform the procedure.

'One of the most difficult things about the job is the unsociable working hours,' Sandra explains, *'9-5 doesn't mean 9-5 in a beauty salon, it often means 8-6, or 8-7, as you have to prepare at the start of the day, and clean up at the end.'*

09:00

At 09:00, Sandra has her first treatment. She welcomes her client into the salon, offers her a drink and then takes her into the treatment room. After communicating with the client to ensure she has all of the correct details, and affirming the details and type of procedure that will take place, Sandra begins. The treatment involves an eyebrow wax and shaping, which should take a maximum of fifteen minutes to complete.

During this treatment, Sandra begins a discussion with her client. Sandra's client has recently undergone a fairly messy divorce, and as the conversation develops, gets fairly upset. Sandra speaks to her in a calm and soothing voice, acting as a therapist with whom the client feels comfortable to talk. She fetches her a drink, finishes the treatment and then allows her time to sit and talk about her issue. All of this means that while the procedure should have taken 15 minutes, it in fact took 40, and the treatment ends at 09:40, instead of 09:15.

10:00

After spending 20 minutes preparing the treatment room for her next client, who is 10 minutes late, Sandra begins her next appointment at 10:10. This treatment is 2 hours long, and includes a facial and a pedicure. These are some of the most popular treatments available in a beauty salon, and will be performed anywhere you work.

In order to perform the facial treatment, Sandra must go through several different steps:

- **Consultation**. Sandra begins the facial with a consultation. This requires the client to fill in a form that enquires about: diet, skin care, consumption of water, any current drugs or medication you prescribe to and any other products you are currently using.

- **Cleansing**. Sandra wraps the client's hair in a towel or head-band, and then cleanses the skin, using cotton pads and wipes.

- **Skin Analysis**. Sandra uses a magnifying lamp to examine the client's skin type. She is looking for signs that indicate the client's skin type: oily, sensitive, dry; and skin condition: black-heads, whiteheads, acne and dehydration. Based on what she sees during this examination, she will consult with the client and then decide on the appropriate products and treatment for the client's skin.

- **Steaming**. Sandra follows up her analysis, by using a facial steamer on the client. This relaxes the skin, which helps to soften blackheads and whiteheads for treatment extraction. During the steaming process, Sandra also uses a mechanical exfoliant to remove dead skin cells from the face.

- **Extraction**. After consulting with the client, Sandra begins the process of extracting blackheads and whiteheads from the face. This should take no longer than ten minutes, but the client experiences some discomfort from the initial technique that Sandra uses, with tools. Therefore Sandra switches meth-ods, using cotton buds between her fingers, to coax the debris from the follicle.

- **Massage**. Sandra then delivers a facial massage, using practiced techniques, to stimulate and relax the client's facial muscles.

- **Masking**. Following this, Sandra applies a facial mask to the client. In this instance Sandra uses a peel off mask, and while waiting for it take effect, delivers a relaxing scalp massage.

During the pedicure, Sandra accidentally smudges her client's toenail. Whilst she would normally have a space between treatments at this point, in order to fix her error, Sandra must cut some time out from this break. In total the treatment takes 2 hours and 15 minutes to complete. Her next treatment begins at 1pm.

13:00

At 13:00, a joint appointment has been booked. This is for a husband and wife, as a promotional package. Sandra takes care of the wife, while another therapist performs treatment on the man. Similarly to the previous treatment, Sandra must perform a facial. This takes 1 hour and 30 minutes to complete. The client in particular has just come in for what is called 'a pamper session' and therefore is not particularly talkative, she just wants to relax. Often, this can be beneficial for a therapist like Sandra. It gives her time to collect her own thoughts without chatting for an hour or so. The only downside is that it is physical work, and by the end of this treatment, Sandra is extremely tired. Following the treatment she successfully promotes and sells two skin products to the client.

14:30

At 14:30, Sandra is booked to perform a half hour waxing treatment. This treatment involves waxing the client's lip, chin and eyebrows. Sandra's client has recently undergone a back operation, so she takes extra care to make sure the client is as comfortable as possible prior to the treatment. This, combined with the fact that the client's back operation is an interesting point of discussion, means that the treatment runs over by 10 minutes. Sandra is scheduled to have her lunch break from 15:00 to 15:30, and now only has 20 minutes instead of 30.

15:30

Sandra begins her next treatment at 15:30. This is another waxing treatment, but this time the client wants a 'Hollywood', a treatment that involves removing all of the client's pubic hair. This takes approximately half an hour to complete, and is a procedure that many aspiring beauty therapists are nervous to perform, particularly when the client has arrived in an unsanitary condition. Sandra, however, has no issue,

'You get used to it', she says, 'As long as the client is clean, after you've done 4 or 5 it becomes as normal as any other treatment.'

In order to perform a Hollywood Wax, Sandra takes the following steps:

- After offering the client a drink, Sandra shows them into a private room, before leaving the client alone to remove their clothes, from the waist down, and get comfortable on a treatment couch covered in sheets or paper.

- First, Sandra applies talcum powder to the skin, to ensure that the hot wax won't stick.

- Next, Sandra dips her wooden stick into the pot of hot wax, and spreads the wax over the skin, ensuring that the client is comfortable with the temperature of the wax.

- Sandra then presses a cloth strip to the hot wax over the skin, so that the cloth, hair and wax stick together.

- Sandra waits a few seconds for the wax to cool, and then pulls the strip in the opposite direction to the hair growth. This uproots the hairs. In this particular treatment, the client felt extremely uncomfortable after the first strip, so Sandra spends some time uprooting smaller areas, one at a time. She repeats this until the entire pubic area is bare.

- Sandra follows up the waxing by removing any stray hairs with tweezers, or trimming the remaining area. She then applies lotion to cool and sooth the affected area.

- After checking the client is comfortable, happy with the treatment result and has the necessary aftercare advice, Sandra books another appointment for the client, in 3 weeks time. This treatment often becomes a regular procedure for clients, who will return every 3 to 4 weeks for a repeat. It is therefore important for Sandra to build up a rapport, particularly with new customers, as clients will ideally return to see the same therapist for their repeat treatment. For new customers, it can be an uncomfortable experience, and therefore by building familiarity the treatment will be easier for both client and therapist.

16:00

From 16:00 to 17:00, Sandra is booked to perform another facial. Unfortunately, during the treatment, the steaming machine breaks. This delays the treatment by several minutes, whilst Sandra makes the necessary adjustments to fix it. This means that the treatment finishes at 17:20. The client does not want to talk much during the treatment, and is unhappy with the delay, as this means she is late for her next appointment. Sandra apologises sincerely, and attempts to negotiate a follow up appointment, but the client leaves without re-booking.

17:00

Now that her treatments for the day are finished, Sandra must begin the process of preparing the salon for the next day. Her duties include:

- Counting the end of day takings
- Emptying the bins
- Putting towels and treatment sheets in the washing machine
- Tumble-drying the towels and treatment sheets after washing
- Washing up cups, plates and surfaces

- Sweeping up, particularly following exfoliation treatment that can leave the floor gritty and dirty

- Ensuring all machines and lights are switched off

We will now move onto our second salon expert, who runs her own salon, and therefore has more responsibility than Sandra.

Julie

08:15

Julie begins her day at 8:15. Before arriving at the salon, or on the way to work, her first task is to get into contact with the suppliers or representatives of the products that her salon promotes and sells, to organise a delivery or pickup. Recognising and organising the intake of these products is a vital part of managing a beauty salon, as local beauty salons can live and die on these sales.

08:30

At 8:30, Julie arrives at the salon. With the help of her team, which today will consist of 4 other therapists, she prepares and sets up the salon for the day ahead. With five different therapists present, each member of staff will be using a different area of the salon, and therefore it is important that every room is prepared for treatment. Julie checks and confirms her appointments in the reception book, and then prepares her own treatment room.

09:00

Julie has her first client at 09:00. This is a regular client, whom she will treat until 10:30. She will perform 3 different treatments on the client: a HD eyebrow shape, a half-leg wax and a neck, back and shoulder massage. Julie begins with the eyebrow shaping.

A 'HD Brow' treatment is a five step procedure that focuses on altering the shape and design of the eyebrows. It is a treatment utilised by many celebrity stylists, and has become increasingly popular within salons as a result.

- First Julie performs an assessment and consultation with the client, confirming the desired shape, colouring and thickness of the brows. Using her experience, she then discusses with the client whether their particular wants are suitable for their skin type and shape face. Upon coming to a suitable conclusion in all categories, Julie begins the treatment.

- The next step involves tinting the brows. First Julie sanitises her client's hands, to ensure they are clean for the later threading process. She then cleanses the brow area. Following this, she chooses from a selection of colours, and tints both the eyebrows and the surrounding hairs. She leaves the tint on several minutes, to ensure it won't fade, and then removes any excess product from the surrounding area.

- Step three is to mark, measure and then wax the brows. Julie uses an eyebrow marker to highlight the areas where she will take the hair from, in order to gain the desired shape. She draws a line around the areas that will be untouched, and then waxes above and below the lines she has drawn.

- Following this, Julie begins the process of threading the eyebrows. This is done to blend in any finer hairs, to the tint and shape that has already been achieved. It is softer and more comfortable for the client than tweezing, and involves rolling a cotton or polyester thread over the areas of unwanted hair. The client holds her eyes shut while this is performed.

- Julie then uses a pencil and palette to finish the look. Eventually the hair will be trained to grow to the desired shape, but for now Julie uses a makeup pencil to fill in any gaps. The customer in question is having her first HD treatment, and therefore she will be required to return in 6 weeks for further work. Julie then plucks and brushes the brows to remove any stray hairs, ensures the client is happy with the results, and moves onto the wax and massage sections of the treatment.

10:30

At 10:30, Julie has a reflexology treatment. This is a treatment involving the feet, hands or ears, and sometimes all three. It is used as a relaxation technique to release tension and restore balance and harmony to the body. In this particular instance, Julie chooses to focus solely on the client's feet.

- Firstly, the client removes her socks and shoes. She then sits and Julie washes her feet in warm water, before bringing them up to chest level.

- Julie then begins a consultation with the client, in relation to any rashes, bunions, sores, leg wounds or feet pain, which could affect or slow down the treatment. It is important that Julie knows all of these details as it is her aim to bring the client maximum comfort and relaxation.

- Following the consultation, Julie works with gentle pressure to massage and relax all areas of the client's foot, to try and produce an internal, positive reaction from the rest of the client's body. The client has been suffering from migraines, and therefore Julie pays particular attention to the migraine points on the toes. This process lasts for half an hour.

- After completing the procedure, Julie finishes by gently stroking the client's foot, offering them a glass of water and then allowing them a period of recovery time. A reflexology session can provoke a number of different physical and mental reactions from clients, and in this case the client has been left feeling both light headed and thirsty. When the client has finished recovering from the treatment, Julie arranges a follow up appointment for 3 weeks' time.

11:10

At 10 past 11, Julie has a scheduled appointment with a newer member of staff. In this meeting she discusses any worries that the staff member might have, potential targets and future training that she would like the staff member to undertake. This meeting goes well, and serves as an appraisal. Both Julie and the new staff member are left feeling positive. As manager of a salon, it is important that Julie nurtures and develops young therapists, so that they can better their skills and improve their techniques on her clients. This meeting takes half an hour.

11:40

From 11:40 till 13:00, Julie has no clients. She therefore uses this time to take her lunch break, and arrange and sort stock. As Julie is the only therapist not performing treatment during this period, she also works the reception, and checks back with any clients who have rang/left messages to book future appointments.

13:00

Julie's next appointment takes 1 hour to complete. She has a 10 minute Electrolysis treatment, and another HD Brow shaping. Electrolysis is a hair removal procedure, where individual hairs are removed from selected, small areas of the body. The treatment works by inserting minute probes into the hair follicle, transmitting energy to the root. The hair is then taken, but not pulled out. This is a less painful, and more effective method than simply plucking. Customers usually agree to a course of treatment, over 5 or 6 sessions, rather than simply having one. The client in question is receiving her second treatment.

14:00

At 14:00, Julie has another Electrolysis treatment, and a hot lip wax. This proves to be an extremely eventful appointment, as upon chatting with the client, Julie discovers that she has recently lost her mother. The client gets very emotional during this session, and needs to take a break. Julie acts as a caring therapist, fetches the client a drink, and sits and talks with her for a while until she is ready to carry on the procedure. The appointment is scheduled to finish at half past 2, but lasts until 10 to 3. Unfortunately for Julie, she has another appointment booked for 14:40, and the client has arrived early. The treatment itself involves a lip, chin and eyebrow wax; therefore Julie instructs one of the free therapists currently available, to perform the first half of the treatment, and she will take over when she is finished. Thus she uses her excellent management skills to negotiate a difficult situation, and ensure that all her clients are happy, and not kept waiting for longer than they need to be.

15:20

Julie finishes her half of the aforementioned treatment at 20 past 3. After successfully promoting and selling three skin products to a customer who has walked in, she is finished with treatments for the day. As the manager of the salon, she now has to perform a variety of admin tasks. Her first job is to check and answer the salon emails. These can relate from customer bookings, to potential new services, advertising, job application forms and stock suppliers. As a salon owner, Julie also has to keep up to date with potential new treatments and services, developments in the beauty world and visit trade shows and markets. She must use her judgement to decide on which of these services is most appropriate for her salon, and whether to invest in selected upgrades or current products. This entire process takes her until 16:00 to complete.

16:00

From 16:00 till 17:00, Julie deals with the promotional aspect of her salon. Her salon has its own Facebook page, which Julie uses to interact with her customers. This is an extremely useful tool, as customers are more vocal via the internet about specific needs and ideas, and Julie can utilise this to deal with suggestions and complaints. She also uses this page to promote deals, products and services that might attract new or returning customers. On her page today, there are two complaints, and several more enquiries. The two complaints come from customers who Julie knows have not been booked into the salon at any point, and therefore are false. She answers in a calm and professional manner, to ensure potential customers are not put off by negative activity on her page, and apologises regardless, since it is important to promote the message that 'the customer is always right'.

Julie follows this up by answering the rest of the customer enquiries on her page, promoting 3 new products that will shortly be available at the salon, and posting information about new and upcoming deals and vouchers the salon will be offering within the next fortnight. 1 of the enquiries is in regards to a potential apprenticeship. She messages the asker of this privately, giving her an email address to contact so that details and a meeting can be arranged.

17:00

At 17:00, the salon closes. Julie and her team spend the next hour and a half tidying up the salon; sweeping, washing, tumble-drying, ensuring the end of day takings match up, checking the appointments for the following day.

20:00

At least one day a week, Julie spends an hour and a half of her evening checking the salon accounts and readying wages for monthly payment. She also prepares training programmes for apprentice staff, and appraisal questions for recently employed therapists. This takes her almost an hour and a half to complete.

Hopefully the two above examples should give you a good idea of what to expect from both working in, and running, a beauty salon. As we have explained, it is a physically demanding task, which requires great patience and people skills. Below you will find our list of top tips, in order to succeed at working in a salon.

- **Stay positive.** One of the most important elements of working in a salon, is to provide a happy and positive atmosphere in which customers can feel comfortable and relaxed. You must be prepared to put your own troubles aside, to help customers with their own.

- **Time management.** Be prepared to take time out of your own breaks, and reorganise your schedule, in order to accommodate customer needs.

- **Keep up to date with new treatments.** The beauty industry is constantly changing, and as a therapist you will be expected to learn and adapt to new procedures that your salon will introduce. The internet, beauty forums and magazines, are a great way to do this.

- **Practice your promotional skills.** An important, and little known, part of being a beauty therapist is in upselling products to customers. The more product you sell, the more likely the salon is to promote you. Your communicational ability will be key to this.

CHAPTER 8

Mobile Beauty Therapist

The next route we will explore, is that of a mobile beauty therapist. Mobile beauty therapists travel to clients homes, delivering treatment that would normally be found in a salon. They work independently, within the confines of a particular area. Mobile beauty treatments are becoming increasingly popular in the industry today; both the 'come to you' element of the role, and the fact that they are not burdened by the financial cost of renting or paying for a premises, means that mobile beauticians can offer their service at competitive prices. The US in particular has embraced this premise, and it is estimated that up to 1 in 4 beauty treatments in the country are now performed within client's homes. The UK is beginning to follow a similar trend, as mobile beauty therapists become more and more popular.

So why become a mobile beauty therapist? What are the advantages and disadvantages? We asked our team of experts to elaborate on the biggest pros and cons that they have found when performing the role.

Advantages

- Mobile beauty therapists can pick and choose which hours they work, therefore making it easier to work around being a Mum, or carer.

- As an independent business owner, you take all of the profits.

- You rarely have 'no shows', as the appointment itself is dependent on you turning up.

- Once you've built up a large enough client base, you can start performing some treatments from home.

- The work is very social, you get to know people much more intimately in the comfort of their own home. You will find yourself performing treatments in many different locations, such as gardens, bedrooms, living rooms. You may have to answer the door for the customer during treatment, which can be an interesting experience, and may meet their children or pets.

- There is more freedom than working in a salon, you can choose what you do and don't do.

Disadvantages

- The time it takes to travel between locations, and being in a car for so much of the day. You can also never predict the traffic, which sometimes leads to late appointments. Fuel costs are also extremely expensive, particularly when doing town appointments, where the traffic is very stop/start.

- The physical side of the job. Transporting heavy equipment from your car to the client's home, and back again, can be exhausting work. This is particularly difficult if the client has several flights of stairs, and very often won't offer to help you.

- Clients often delay the treatment to perform household tasks such as washing, ironing, cooking or cleaning, which sets you back for the day.

- Clients sometimes forget that they have booked the treatment. If they aren't home, then you are left waiting around for them to return, whereas if you worked in a salon, you would be able to busy yourself doing something else/preparing for the next treatment.

- If you aren't getting bookings, you aren't making money. There is no salon wage to fall back on.

Getting started

Starting your own business can be an extremely scary process. Unlike simply working in a salon, here you are working independently and if the business does not succeed, you are the person who will lose out. If you are off sick, or physically unable to perform treatments, then there is nobody to cover your pay. Many mobile beauticians start by working in a salon, and then use the skills they have picked up from this role to work independently. In order to work as a mobile beauty therapist, you must be highly experienced and capable of performing treatments, as unlike working in a salon, there is nobody there to teach you the correct procedure. Therefore the first thing you need are qualifications. These are no different to those of a regular salon worker; you will require a Level 3 NVQ or SVQ certificate in beauty therapy, or equivalent, or an ITEC Level 3 Diploma in advanced beauty therapy. If you are someone who really wants to make the leap, direct from either college or a salon apprenticeship, then there are plenty of training courses available for you to enhance your skills, prior to taking the commitment. Organisations such as Cidesco offer centres and courses that aim to teach and advance your knowledge in the subject, and therefore enhance your treatment procedure.

You will also need a reliable, and spacious form of transport. As a mobile beauty therapist, you will be spending most of the day in the car travelling between different treatments. Therefore it is essential you have a valid driving license and a reliable car or van. A van would be particularly useful in this instance, as it would provide room for you to stock and transport all of your supplies and equipment. When you arrive at the location chosen for treatment, you will be expected to move most of the equipment from your car to the client's house, and then back again. This can include heavy treatment couches, tables and machinery, and therefore it is important you are in good physical shape.

Finally, you will need to pay for public liability costs, which cover both yourself and your client, obtain a license to practice from your local authority, and pay for insurance costs. Depending on where you live, you may receive your license to practice for free, or have to pay a small fee. Contact your local authority for specific details on the cost of this, and how to obtain it. There are many different options available for mobile beauty therapists in terms of insurance. Signing up for The British Association of Beauty Therapy and Cosmetology, or BABTAC, can be extremely useful. They offer insurance packages and deals to their members, along with the license to use the BABTAC logo on your personal website or promotional material. This will only enhance your reputation, and draw potential customers in. You will also need to pay for professional indemnity insurance, in case a client decides to make a claim against you.

Once you have the recognised qualifications, insurance, a valid driving license, a reliable form of transport, and you feel you are experienced enough to begin working independently, there are several things to consider:

Market Research

Before beginning your mobile beauty business, it is extremely important to research the area you will be conducting your business in. You also need to set yourself guidelines on how far you are willing to travel. Timing is a crucial factor when working as an independent therapist, and therefore it is a good idea, particularly initially, to keep your target area local and small. If you are travelling huge distances every single day then you will not only lose money on fuel, but there are likely to be delays between clients. After you have decided upon your locational boundaries, you must assess the competeviness of the area in which you are operating. Look at the type of treatments that your competitors offer and the price they charge. A good way to do this, is to use either the internet or yellow pages, to see just how many independent therapists operate in your area. Even arranging a treatment from one of these potential competitors, in the comfort of your own home, would be useful. You will be able to see how your competition operates and how you can better this. As a mobile therapist, you need to find a unique selling point which differentiates you from your competition.

Types of Treatment

Once you have performed your market research, you need to decide which types of treatment you will offer. When starting out, it is a good idea to keep your treatment bracket fairly small. Whether you trained in a salon, or achieved your qualification through a college course, think about what types of treatments you performed best at, and which ones you enjoyed doing the most. You should use your market research to gage the popularity and competitiveness of treatments in the area. For example, if your research shows that there are large amounts of nail salons and independent nail technicians/specialists within the area, then it would be unwise to specialise in this yourself. Initially, you should try to find a treatment that is unique, stands out from your competitors and will therefore attract customers to your new business. Consider more advanced treatments that you are qualified to perform, such as Indian head massage or Reflexology, and make them an integral part of your service list.

Equipment and costs

When you have decided which treatments you will perform, you will then need to purchase the equipment necessary for these treatments. The first thing most mobile beauty therapists invest in, is a comfortable and portable treatment couch. These can be folded up, placed in your car or van, and then moved back and forth between your vehicle and the client's home. You will also need to purchase a wax pot, manicure tables and tools, pedicure tools and eyebrow shaping and tinting equipment, depending on the services you choose to offer.

Combined with the cost of a potential new vehicle, and future fuel costs, this can all seem like a pricey investment. However, you should consider that once you have purchased all of the equipment, the overhead costs will be very little. When deciding which equipment to purchase, work out the financial implications of how much you expect to charge for each treatment, which treatments you expect to be the most popular and how much revenue you will make within the first 3 months. It is a good idea, when setting your treatment prices, to maintain a minimum treatment charge, usually around £10-£20. If a client only wants a service that costs £5, then it is unlikely you will be making any money on the treatment, and therefore will be wasting your time.

As our expert tells us, the mobile beauty industry can be extremely lucrative:

'The pay is very good as you have very few overheads due to the mobile nature of the job, just fuel and replaceable equipment; make-up pencils, wax strips, etc. Potentially I can earn between £100 and £200 a day, sometimes more.'

Provided you get enough customers, and as long you can afford it, investing in high quality equipment will only benefit you in the long run. You should take the same attitude towards advertising and promotional costs. The word of mouth nature of the industry means that just one really high quality advert can kick start your business.

If you are worried about the money, and feel you might struggle to pay for the equipment and costs, there are a number of options available:

A business loan

In reality, the likelihood of you managing to secure a business loan is slim. Banks are highly experienced in start-up business and realize that only a few ever make it past the first few years of trading. Before they consider giving you a business loan they will want to see how much you are prepared to invest yourself, which in most cases will be nothing. However, if you are in a position where you can part fund your business loan then there is more chance of you obtaining investment.

Venture Capitalists

A venture capitalist is someone who invests capital in a business venture. Conventionally, venture capitalists are looking for a higher rate of return than might be given by more traditional investments such as a bank loan. This will normally be in the form of shares in return for their investment. Naturally you will feel reluctant to part with your shares but it is worth bearing in mind the following:

When you start out with a new business idea or venture, your 100% shareholding will be worth next to nothing. If you do not get the right kind of investment, those 100% shares might still not amount to much three years down the line. However, if you give up 40% of your shares to a venture capitalist for a £200,000 investment, the 60% that you then have might be worth a lot more than the 100% in three years time!

In addition, bear in mind that with most investors you will also be gaining their experience and knowledge. After all, they will want to see their investment flourish just as much as you do.

Business Angels

Business angels are usually wealthy individuals who are prepared to invest in high-growth businesses in return for equity or shares. Some business angels invest on their own, whereas others do so as part of a network, syndicate group or investment club. In addition to money, business angels often make their own skills, experience and contacts available to the company, which is obviously of benefit to you. With a bank loan or a loan from a friend or company there is more pressure on you to make the business work.

Business angels typically invest in businesses with an investment need of between £10,000 and £250,000 - most initial investments are less than £75,000. The advantage of using a business angel is that they often make an investment decision quickly, without complex assessments. However, you will still need to draw up a professional business plan. Most business angels are also likely to have local knowledge, as they tend to focus their investments within a small geographical area. Again this can be advantageous to you and your new business.

The disadvantage of business angels is that they don't make investments very regularly and may not be actively looking for an opportunity, so they may be difficult to find. While you may decide to approach an agency to help you with this, business angels will place a lot of emphasis on your relationship with them and how well you can work together directly. Tracking down the right investor may take longer than expected and can typically take several months. The British Business Angels Association (BBAA) will direct you to local and appropriate business angel networks and provide guidance with preparing and presenting your business proposal.

www.ukbusinessangelsassociation.org.uk

Some business angels could also have their investment funds matched by the government under its Enterprise Capital Funds (ECFs) scheme. ECFs targeted at Small and Medium-sized Enterprises (SMEs) are under development, and will only win government approval if they clearly show how they are targeting SMEs.

In effect, ECFs are commercial funds that invest a combination of private and public money against a share of equity in small high-growth businesses seeking up to £2 million of equity finance. You can find out more about the ECF scheme here:

www.capitalforenterprise.gov.uk

Understanding gross, net profit, balance sheets and profit & loss accounts

Before you approach any form of potential financer, have a thorough understanding of gross and net profit. It would also be handy to have a basic understanding of a balance sheet.

Gross Profit is calculated by deducting the cost of goods sold from the net sales figure. The calculation of the gross profit takes place in the trading account.

Net Profit is the excess of gross profit over expenditure. It is calculated in the profit and loss account by deducting all business expenditure from the gross profit.

The importance of quality customer service

As soon as you start your business, and especially when you begin trading, make sure your customer service is of the highest standard. In order to build a successful business you will need to build a good name. A successful business cannot be built on repeat business alone, therefore it is essential that you obtain new customers. Naturally this can be done via advertising, but the best form of advertising is free and is achieved via 'word of mouth'.

A satisfied and happy customer is likely to recommend you to one other person, whereas an unhappy customer will tell ten other people about their bad experience with your company. Therefore, the only effective way to build a good reputation is to build quality customer service.

Business Bank Account

You will need a business bank account if you are running a business. You simply can't survive without one. It is the focal point of your business finances, showing all the financial transactions of your business. A business bank account is where you pay money in, pay suppliers and your workforce, draw out petty cash and complete all of the other essential financial transactions involved in running a business.

If you're a sole trader, this will keep your business account separate from your personal finances. Whatever type of business you run, it will be essential for calculating tax. A business bank account can in some cases give you access to support, advice and finance. You will need to decide which bank to use. Before you start comparing different banks it's worth knowing the products and services they may offer.

Bank facilities for business owners

- **Deposits:** Paying in cash and cheques.

- **Withdrawals:** Taking out cash through an ATM or at a branch.

- **Payment by cheque:** Use of a business chequebook, which can sometimes be personalised with your company logo.

- **Automatic money transfers:** Direct debits and direct credits.

- **Night safe:** For depositing money when the bank is closed.

- **Balance enquiry and statements:** For keeping track of your finances.

- **Company debit card:** This will debit an amount immediately from your business account. In most cases the transactions are free and there is no annual fee.

- **Company credit card:** A charge card (such as Barclaycard or MasterCard) that can be issued to key members of staff. Repayments are made monthly from your business current account (usually interest free credit). There is usually a fee per transaction, an annual fee or both.

- **Overdraft and loan facilities:** Short-term financing, subject to an application procedure. May also provide access to the Government-backed Small Firm Loan

- **Asset finance:** Leasing and hire purchase facilities to enable you to buy equipment.

- **Factoring and invoice discounting:** Short-term borrowing against the value of unpaid invoices.

- **Commercial mortgage:** Funding to help you buy a business property. Often up to 80% of the purchase can be financed by the bank.

- **Deposit accounts:** A lot of banks have business deposit accounts with higher interest than a current account for any reserve funds your business may have.

- **Merchant services:** If you want to accept credit and debit card payments from customers, you will need a merchant account. This is provided by a bank but to get one you will often need two years' trading history and audited accounts. Once set-up, you will be charged an annual fee plus a percentage of every transaction.

- **Insurance:** The larger banks will often offer their customers insurance cover for business interruption, health, loan repayments and more.

- **Support:** Most of the larger banks offer resources and support to help you run your business. For example, you may be assigned a relationship manager who will offer business advice. The bank may also provide seminars, educational literature or bookkeeping software.

- **Introductory offers:** The main banks offer special introductory offers to start-ups. This is usually a period of free banking for 12-24 months.

An Accountant - Do I need one?

An accountant will be another source of business advice when you first start running your own business. They will be able to advise you on your business plan and the tax issues of registering a new business. Some accountants offer bookkeeping services but if they don't or if you wish to handle this yourself, you can get help with setting up manual or computerised bookkeeping systems. Most importantly, you need an accountant to assist on things like whether it is necessary to register for VAT or PAYE and the procedures involved.

An accountant will also give you financial advice and help with budgeting, cash flow and credit control, in addition to up-to-date information on any general or legal enquiries.

As your business grows

Whether you are starting up or a growing business, an accountant can advise you on the best way to arrange additional finance without putting your business at risk. Remember, an accountant isn't just there to help you manage your money. Once you have the finance in place there needs to be some control to ensure growth of your business is handled in the right way. Many of your concerns will be financial - adequate working capital, good stock control, invoicing and so on – so an experienced accountant's advice will be invaluable in such matters. Also, an accountant will be on top of all the current taxation issues. Taxation is a large business expense and an accountant can effectively minimise these costs.

VALE ADDED TAX (VAT)

If you're in business, you must register for VAT if your VAT taxable turnover for the previous twelve months is more than £79,000. This figure is known as the VAT registration threshold. The threshold changes - usually once a year announced in the Budget - so you should regularly check your turnover against the current threshold.

You must also register for VAT if either of the following applies:

- you think your VAT taxable turnover may go over the threshold in the next 30 days alone

- you take over a VAT-registered business as a going concern

VAT quarterly returns must be completed and sent to HM Customs and Excise along with any payment due. The VAT forms are very simple - just a single page, in fact - and usually work in the company's favour. This is because although you must pay VAT on any income generated, you can claim back VAT paid on some goods and services, such as office supplies, vehicle servicing, fuel and so on. So the extra accounting is definitely worth it and even companies whose turnover is less than the VAT limit can still register voluntarily. Not all products and services attract the standard VAT rate, so it's worth contacting your local HMC&E office to request one of their introductory videos, which will explain the basics of VAT accounting.

Keep yourself up to date with the latest VAT information and rates by listening to the Budget. This will be done by your accountant/ bookkeeper but it is good for you and your business to be aware of this information. Remember you are expected to account for every business-related penny spent and you are expected to show each month's profit/loss and income/expenditure in sufficient detail so that the tax can be clearly calculated.

Accountancy software

Buying an accountancy software package can slash the amount of time and effort you put into managing your finances. In the early stages you could use the services of a freelance bookkeeper or your accountant, as mentioned above, who will have the software and keep your books up to date on a monthly basis for a fee.

Marketing

As with any business, marketing and promotion will be crucial to your success. You might consider starting your own website, at a small cost, or using social media such as Facebook and Twitter to promote your services to the wider world. It is extremely important that as a business owner, you engage and interact with your clients. This will enhance your reputation and help you to build up a dedicated client base. Facebook in particular can be used to create promotions, deals and special offers, which will generate interest for your company name. You should also use friends-of- friends and family, to encourage new customers to give your services a try. Word of mouth is an extremely effective tool, as one of our experts explains.

'I've always worked solely on word of mouth. It was fairly easy to pick up new clients from the start, as the parents at my youngest daughters school were all extremely interested. Once several of them gave my service a try, they spread the word to their friends, and the business grew from there.'

Whereas salon workers operate from the confines of an established treatment room, as a mobile technician you are being invited into your client's home, and therefore it is extremely important you engage with them on a personal level. Reaching out to potential clients via Facebook and Twitter can be a great way to start off your marketing campaign. You might also consider paying for beauty business cards, and promotional leaflets, to further enhance the professionalism of your product.

Another option available, is to use Google Pay per Click Advertising.

Pay-per-click Advertising

Pay-per-click (PPC) advertising was first introduced by Yahoo.com back in the early 2000's. Although Yahoo was the first company to introduce PPC advertising, it was Google who really dominated the market by making their systems both highly effective and functional, but also relevant to what people were searching for – this still stands true today. 'Relevance' is the key to PPC advertising, and Google certainly got this bit right. The latest figures distributed reveal that over 80% of traffic searches are handled by Google. The remainder of traffic is spread about amongst the other search engine sites such as Yahoo (Bing), Ask and MSN.

What makes this great for you as an online advertiser, is that you can get literally thousands of 'relevant' visitors to your website within seconds. Of course, there are a number of pitfalls when using PPC advertising, but if you take the time to learn the system, then you can make an absolute fortune in the process.

Keyword searches

People who search for goods or information online will type in a word or a phrase into the search engine. Once they click 'search', then they will be provided with hundreds or thousands, and some-times millions of pages of 'relevant' websites. These websites are provided in order of most relevance and Google will use its unique **PageRank** system to achieve this. The websites that appear on the natural rankings of Google get most of the traffic for free. Therefore, there is a great incentive to get your website to appear in these free rankings.

Taking into account all of the above information, it is vitally import-ant that you choose your 'keywords and phrases' very carefully. In addition to the natural search rankings that Google creates, you will also notice that there are a number of 'sponsored results' at the very top of the page and also on the right hand side of the search engine page. These are what are called 'paid for advertising', or PPC as we better know them.

Every time a person clicks on your advert, you have to pay for it, re-gardless of whether they buy anything or not! Therefore, there's a lot more to online advertising than simply getting traffic to your website. In very basic terms, you will decide how much you are prepared to pay every time a person clicks through your advert. This will very much depend on how much your product or service is selling for. For example, a person who is selling a DVD for £10 is certainly not going to bid £10 per click as they will be out of business before the end of the day. They are far more likely to bid something like £0.10 per click.

Now here's the trick. In order to pay less for your adverts and each time a person clicks through on it, you MUST make your advert relevant. This can be achieved in a number of ways:

1. Choose a domain name that matches, or is similar to, the search term.

2. Make sure you include the search term in your advert - Google will make relevant domains and search terms bold so that they stand out.

3. Use 'capitalisation' in your adverts. Again, these will allow the advert to stand out from the rest.

The more your advert stands out from the rest, the more people will click through on it. If more people are clicking through on your advert, then it must mean your website is relevant to the search term.

In order to help you get the most from PPC advertising, here are a few great tips:

- It is worth considering paying a professional company to set up your campaign for you if your budget will stretch. The reason for this is that you can end up wasting lots of money on clicks that will not convert and a professional company will be able to test your adverts and keywords for you.

- When you start advertising using PPC, set your daily budget quite low. This will allow you to test the market and see whether or not your product or service actually converts. If you are getting lots of visitors to your website but none of them are buying or interacting then there may be an issue with your website or service.

- Add **negative keywords** to your campaign. Negative keywords can help you to reach the most interested customers, reduce your costs and increase your return on investment (ROI). When you add negative keywords your ad won't show to people searching for those terms or visiting sites that contain those terms. With negative keywords, you can:

- Prevent your ad from showing to people searching for or visiting websites about things that you don't offer.

- Show your ads to people who are more likely to click them.

- Reduce costs by excluding keywords where you might be spending money but not getting a return.

- When you select negative keywords, you'll want to choose search terms that are similar to your keywords, but signal that people are looking for a different product.

Marketing

As with any business, marketing and promotion will be crucial to your success. You might consider starting your own website, at a small cost, or using social media such as Facebook and Twitter to promote your services a wider audience. It is extremely important that as a business owner, you engage and interact with your clients. This will enhance your reputation and help you to build up a dedicated client base. Facebook in particular can be used to create promotions, deals and special offers, which will generate interest for your company name. You should also use friends-of-friends and family, to encourage new customers to give your services a try. Word of mouth is an extremely effective tool, as one of our experts explains:

'I've always worked solely on word of mouth. It was fairly easy to pick up new clients from the start, as the parents at my youngest daughters school were all extremely interested. Once several of them gave my service a try, they spread the word to their friends, and the business grew from there.'

Whereas salon workers operate from the confines of an established treatment room, as a mobile technician you are being invited into your client's home, and therefore it is extremely important you engage with them on a personal level. Reaching out to potential clients via Facebook and Twitter can be a great way to start off your marketing campaign. You might also consider paying for beauty business cards, and promotional leaflets, to further enhance the professionalism of your service.

As you can see, starting up as a mobile beautician can be difficult. There are a wide range of activities you must do to prepare for the role, and this can be off-putting for many aspiring therapists. This is why most mobile therapists begin by working in a salon, rather than making the jump straight after their apprenticeship or college course. With this in mind, here at How2Become we have prepared a sample day, taken from the real life experience of one of our experts, to show you exactly what to expect from the role.

Helen is a mobile beauty therapist from Kent. She has been performing the role for ten years, and has an established client base that she regularly treats on a day to day basis. She has two children; the youngest of whom influenced her decision to become a mobile therapist:

'I was working 3 days a week, as a salon therapist in London. When my youngest daughter started school, I decided I didn't want to do it anymore. The travel was too hard. I didn't have a space in own home to treat clients, so I decided to work mobile. It's the best decision I've ever made'.

As a mobile beautician, Helen works from 9-5 most days of the week, depending on how many appointments she has. The below example is one of her recent weekdays.

Helens Day

08:00

Helens day begins at 08:00. After checking her appointment book, ensuring she knows the correct location of each treatment and then ensuring she has the suitable products and equipment stored in the back of her car, she leaves the house at 08:30.

After dropping her children off at school, she is back in her car by 08:50. Her first appointment is at half past 9, but due to traffic from the school run, she arrives 10 minutes late. After apologising sincerely to the sympathetic client, she performs her first treatment. This consists of a short lip, chin and eyebrow wax, which takes around fifteen minutes to complete.

10:00

Helens next appointment is at 10:15. Upon arrival to the house, she discovers that the client is feeding her new baby. This means that for the next twenty minutes, Helen must sit and wait, whilst her client feeds him and gets him to sleep. By the time they finally get round to the treatment, Helen is over half an hour behind schedule. The treatment is a pedicure. In order to perform the pedicure, Helen takes the following steps, on each foot:

- First, she removes any present, old nail polish from the toenails. She uses a licensed, nail polish remover to do this.

- Next, Helen fills the portable basin she has brought with her, with warm soapy water, and instructs the client to place her feet inside. She leaves the feet to soak for ten minutes, which allows any dirt to be removed and for any calluses to soften.

- After drying the client's feet, Helen begins filing the toenails. She uses nippers to remove the underside of the corners, preventing potential pain, and uses a grit-file to round the toenails, so that they are in line with the shape of the toe.

- Once this has been completed, Helen uses cuticle trimmers, to push back and trim the excess skin around the nail. This will better prepare the clients toenails for the painting process. After she has done this, Helen applies a small amount of cuticle oil to the affected area of each toe, to sooth and moisten the skin.

- Next, Helen smooths the top of the nails using a buffing pad, filing down any rough edges or ridges. She then uses a foot paddle to file any calloused skin from the bottom of the foot.

- Following this, Helen begins the massage part of the pedicure. She applies lotion to the bottom of the feet, and slowly works every inch of each foot, the lower legs and the client's toes. Once she has done this, the client puts her feet back into the warm footbath, and Helen uses a spray bottle to remove all traces of the lotion from between her toes, and the tops and bottom of her feet. She then dries the client's foot with a soft towel, and wipes each toenail with a cotton pad, to be sure the nail is free of any remaining product.

- Helen then begins painting the nails. First, she applies a clear, base coat to each toenail, to act as a protective layer against the nail polish, and to give the final layer something to stick to. After agreeing a suitable colour with the client, Helen then administers the decorative paint, and applies another clear, top coat. She chats with the client while the paint dries, ensures she is happy with the final result, and then leaves.

12:30

Helen doesn't have another appointment until 12:30, so following the last client, pops home to get some lunch. This is one of the benefits to working as a mobile therapist. She hoovers, eats lunch and is out of the house by 10 past 12, and on the way to her next appointment. Helen's next appointment is within the town centre, in a block of flats. This means that when she gets there, Helen not only has to park, but to carry her treatment table and equipment up several flights of stairs. By the time she has finished doing this, she is exhausted. The client did not offer to help, and further delays the treatment by finishing her ironing beforehand. Helen, however, still has to perform a lengthy, physical back massage, and therefore this is particularly draining for her. The client also has a child who pesters during the treatment, and at one point knocks over a bottle of massage oil that Helen has brought to the treatment. As she explains, this can be one of the most difficult parts of the process.

'Clients are in their own home, so they feel comfortable to do what-ever they want. There are certain rules in a salon, you adhere to the expectations of the establishment performing the treatment, but as a mobile beauty therapist you don't get any of these benefits. Carting equipment up several flights of stairs can be physically demanding, especially when the client doesn't really help you. I've had friends who switched to performing treatment solely in their own homes, for that exact reason.'

To say thank-you following the treatment, the client leaves Helen with a significant tip, and agrees to a follow up appointment in 2 weeks-time. Helen then has to carry all of her equipment back down the stairs, and back to her car. This time, the client helps her to carry some of the products and bags she has brought. The treatment lasts for 1 hour, and finishes at 13:45.

14:15

Helen's last appointment takes her twenty minutes to get to. The client lives in a country home, some distance away. Upon finding the location, and having a cup of tea with the client, Helen begins her final treatment of the day. This consists of a 'full works' manicure, pedicure, facial, massage and electrolysis. In order to perform the manicure, Helen takes the following steps:

- First, Helen instructs the client to wash, disinfect and then dry her hands. Next, the client moves over to the manicure table Helen has brought with her, and rests her hands flat, on a soft towel. Helen then fills a bowl with warm water.

- Helen uses a cotton pad to remove any old, or still present nail polish on the client's fingernails. Following this, Helen uses an industry approved exfoliant to remove the dead skin from the client's hands and fingers, before drying them off again.

- Helen then begins filing the nails. She uses soft strokes, and an emery board, to file the nails gently down to an acceptable length. After she has finished the filing process, Helen applies cuticle softener to the cuticles and then instructs the client to place her hands in the bowl of warm water.

- Following this, Helen applies hand cream, and massages the hand and wrist area of the client, starting in the centre of the thumb and travelling all the way up to the tips of her fingers. She then washes and sprays the client's fingernails in the warm water, ensuring there is no excess lotion left on either the nails or between the fingers, and dries the hands using a towel.

- Finally, Helen paints the nails of her client, in an agreed colour. She starts off with a clear bottom coat in order to protect the nail, apply the chosen colour and finish with another clear coating. This gives the end product a shining effect, and avoids chipping of the coloured area.

Unfortunately, after completing all of the other treatments, Helen realises she has forgotten to bring the lead for the Electrolysis machine. She apologises sincerely, and agrees to fit the client in for a short Electrolysis appointment tomorrow afternoon. The treatment finishes at 16:00. Following this, Helen must travel back to school, to collect her daughters from after school club, and then get home to prepare dinner.

19:00

From 19:00 till 21:00 every evening, Helen deals with promotion, marketing and preparation for the following day. Firstly, she checks her emails. Sometimes clients will email instead of ringing, to try and book an appointment. Helen has 3 booking requests, for next week. She checks her timetable, and then emails the clients back to confirm their treatments. Next, she logs onto her Facebook Business Page. As a business owner, social media is becoming more and more important in interacting with customers. Helen says that she has had to grasp this concept quickly, in order to keep her business relevant and modern.

'I started my business long before Facebook even existed, so all of my original customers came purely through word of mouth. However, a few years ago I began losing customers to several, new competitors in the area. I've had to adapt and update my methods, and Facebook is a great way to advertise deals and promotions and talk to my customers outside of treatment times. Since I made a business page, my sales figures have been up, and I'm now doing better than I ever was.'

Helen posts a new promotional offer on her Facebook page this evening, available to the first 5 customers who claim it. She then logs onto her Twitter, and posts the same thing. Within half an hour, she has gained 30 likes, and 3 claimants have come forward. Helen messages these customers before switching off the computer. Following this, she checks her appointment book for the following day. Her schedule for tomorrow is:

- 09:30: Lip, chin and eyebrow wax

- 10:30: Reflexology appointment

- 12:00: Indian Head Massage

- 13:30: Facial and back massage

- 14:30: Lip, chin, eyebrow wax and pedicure.

Helen makes sure she has all of the relevant products safely stored in the back of her car, or ready to transport to the car in the morning, has a good idea of where each treatment will take place and how to get there, and then goes to bed.

You should now have a good idea of what to expect, if you are considering a role as a mobile beauty therapist. Below we have listed our top tips, for succeeding in this venture.

- **Stay organised.** As a business owner, organisation is absolutely key. As you have seen from Helen's schedule, you need to prepare in advance of every working day, with maps, products and equipment ready to go. You need to be capable of sorting your own accounts, booking clients in at certain times and working around travel distances.

- **Keep up to date.** This not only applies to using tools such as social media, but maintaining a relevant knowledge of the industry. In order to better your competition, you need to use the internet, visit market shows and read magazines and articles to keep up to date with the latest treatments and procedures.

- **Take part in courses and training.** Prior to starting the business, as a mobile therapist you need to have an advanced and detailed knowledge of every single procedure you will perform. Therefore, after finishing college, or your apprenticeship, it is a great idea to enrol upon and partake in, as many courses as possible. These will boost your knowledge and prepare you better for the challenges ahead. Get in touch with providers such as Cidesco and book your place today.

- **Stay positive.** Remember, just the same as working in a salon, you need to maintain a friendly and positive attitude at all times. There will be challenges, both physical and mental, such as carting heavy equipment around, but as a therapist you must be able to put these issues aside, and provide a friendly service to your customers.

If you would like to find out information on becoming a mobile hairdresser, we have created an in-depth *How to Become a Mobile Hairdresser* guide which you can obtain from **www.How2become.com**

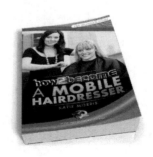

CHAPTER 9

Other options

In this chapter we will explore further options that you might wish to consider, after finishing your beauty degree, or apprenticeship. We will look at what it takes to teach beauty in an institution such as a college, and examine the pros and cons of working on a cruise ship. With the help of our team of experts, we will provide you with all of the information needed to help you make a decision about whether to take one of these career routes.

Teaching Beauty

This is a very popular option for salon therapists. Many therapists spilt their weekly timetable between teaching beauty and working in a salon. In order to teach beauty, the current requirement is that you have a Level 3 Diploma, and a minimum of 3 years commercial experience within the industry. This can vary depending upon where you are applying, as some colleges or institutions may ask for up to 5 years of experience. Typically, beauty lecturers earn up to £30,000 per year, which is similar to most other teaching roles.

If you are someone with a Level 3 Diploma, and several years of experience within the industry, then you are ready to apply. The first step you should take is to ring up your local college, and enquire as to whether there are any places available on their teaching courses. Earning an introductory teaching certificate is a great start for any aspiring teacher. This course will teach you the basics of lesson planning, schemes of work and teaching theory. It will take two years to complete, and as beauty is a vocational and practical field, you will be required to demonstrate practical experience for your assessment. This usually takes place via voluntary work, with the college or establishment itself offering up practical opportunities for aspiring teachers to demonstrate their skills in the classroom environment. You can also contact teachers within your field, and ask to shadow them for a few days. At the end of your teaching course, you will have to complete an A1 assessors award, which will demonstrate that you have the ability to assess and judge beauty students in the classroom environment.

We asked our resident expert what she feels are the biggest advantages, and disadvantages, to teaching beauty:

'The biggest advantages are in the sociable working hours, and the rewarding feeling you get from imparting your hard earned knowledge onto younger students. There are, however, plenty of disadvantages. As with all teaching, the work can be exhausting. You need to be organised, patient and tolerant, especially when it comes to dealing with disruptive students. There are also huge amounts of paperwork to fill in, and you may be required to teach either English or Maths to students who haven't yet got the required GCSE grade.'

With this in mind, let's look at the regular, working day of a beauty lecturer. This will hopefully give you some idea of what to expect, when applying for the role.

Jeanette is a beauty lecturer from Hornchurch. She works from 9 till half past 4 at her local college, on Monday, Tuesday and Friday. She also has her own salon, and barring Sunday, works every other day and most evenings at the shop.

07:15

Jeanette begins her day at 07:15am. After planning her lessons over the weekend, and during her breaks last week, she checks that she has all the necessary material within her teaching folder, gets into her car and heads to work. She arrives at 08:00, and heads into the staff room for a quick meeting with her manager, and the rest of the staff. The meeting takes just under half an hour to complete. The college management and staff are currently readying themselves for an upcoming Ofsted inspection, and therefore good lesson quality is of the highest importance. Jeanette arrives in her classroom at 8:30am, and begins preparing for the opening lesson of the day.

09:00

The first lesson that Jeanette will take, is a Level 2 anatomical class. This lesson will cover areas such as bone structure, muscle function and blood circulation. Jeanette endeavours to make the topic as interesting as possible, by engaging the class in group activities. Prior to the lesson, Jeanette places different words, functions and muscles on each individual desk. The students then move around the room, trying to find the student who has a corresponding word/function to their own. Unfortunately, given it is a Monday morning, Jeanette has some students in the class who are less than happy to be there. She is forced to send two students out, in order to ensure the rest of the lesson runs as smoothly as possible. The class enjoy the group activities Jeanette has planned, and at the end of the session demonstrate their progress by listing the various things they have learned, while Jeanette writes the answers on the board.

10:30

At 10:30, Jeanette has a Level 3 practical class. This is a more advanced group, and the nature of learning is completely different to the previous. In this session, Jeanette will be teaching her Level 3's about Indian Head Massage. She begins with a practical demonstration of how to begin the procedure. Jeanette enjoys teaching Level 3 more than Level 2, because most of the students are interested and engaged with the subject. After finishing her demonstration, the students pair up, pick a treatment couch, and begin practicing the demonstrated techniques on each other. Jeanette moves around the room, observing students and offering advice and tips based on what she sees. After a short period, Jeanette practices the next part of the treatment, on another volunteer, and the students repeat the same process. She does this twice more, before the lesson finishes.

12:30

At 12:30 Jeanette has a Level 2 English class. This is a class designed for students, who have not yet achieved their grade C in English. Jeanette readily admits that this was a huge challenge for her at first:

'I got a C myself, but that was many years ago. I hadn't studied English for several years, so to actually teach the subject was a very daunting prospect. Luckily, the lessons are taught at a very basic, beginner level, so it was easy for me to get used to the topic, and impart knowledge onto the students.'

The lesson consists of activities based around grammar, writing and comprehension. In today's lesson, the students will be engaging in a creative writing exercise. Jeanette puts the students into 6 groups, and gives them each a picture of a well-known fictional or non-fictional character. The job of the students is then to assign motivations, good and bad character qualities, likes and dislikes to each of the figures, before reading this list out to the rest of the class. The rest of the class then have to guess who each of the characters are. Following this, the students must write up a short, creative segment, from their characters perspective, beginning with 'I woke up in the morning'. The group in question is a particularly difficult group to manage, and therefore Jeanette is pleasantly surprised by how smoothly the activity runs. She follows this exercise up by handing out worksheets to the students, which focus on grammar and punctuation. While she has to tell several students to keep the noise down, the lesson goes very well, and Jeanette heads into the lunch period feeling particularly pleased.

14:30

At 14:30, after a 1 hour lunch break, Jeanette has a Level 2 practical class. In this class she will be teaching the students about pedicures. The lesson is in a similar format to the last practical. Jeanette begins by demonstrating the opening stages of the procedure to the students, and then allows them to practice on each other. She then goes round the room, checking and analysing the techniques on display. Similarly to the last group, this is a troublesome class, and Jeanette has some difficulty controlling their behaviour. Particularly since this is a practical exercise, the students must behave in a safe and responsible manner, and at one point Jeanette is forced to take the pedicure tools away from a particular student. Some of the students are also reluctant to perform certain aspects of the treatment, and are uncomfortable touching each other's feet. Jeanette has met many students with similar issues, and gently coaxes them into beginning the treatment. The lesson finishes at 16:30. Jeanette then spends half an hour filling out paperwork, and student behaviour forms, before leaving to go and work at her salon for the next 3 hours.

As you can see from Jeanette's day, a huge part of her role is in controlling the behaviour of her students. Even if you are someone with large amounts of industry experience, imparting this wisdom onto younger, sometimes badly behaved members of the community, is no simple task. With this in mind, we have provided a list of top tips, to help you succeed as a beauty lecturer.

- **Ensure you have enough experience.** Given that many of the lessons consist of taught practical exercises, you must be someone who is well practised in the techniques shown. This is the reason that most colleges require you to have at least 3 years commercial experience within the industry, unlike some teaching qualifications where teachers can come straight from University or College.

- **Stay organised.** A huge part of teaching is in organisational ability. You must be able to lesson plan, organise your time, write up and file paperwork quickly and efficiently. You must be someone who can cope with regular inspection in their workplace, who is willing and ready to adapt and improve their teaching methods.

- **Practice your people skills.** Teaching, in any respect, is a people industry. If you are trained and have experience as a therapist you are more than likely someone who already has a social, friendly attitude; teaching will present you with an altogether new challenge. You must be able to control and negotiate with all kinds of people, some of them rude and badly behaved. You must be disciplined, and firm but fair, to ensure your students respect you and the expertise you can lend them.

Cruise Ship Therapist

If you have read through this guide, and decided by this point, that none of the listed options are suitable for you, we have one final option to suggest. This is an option that many therapists take, and involves working as a beauty therapist on a cruise ship. In order to work as a therapist on board a ship, you will be required to have a minimum of 2 years educational/college experience and a Level 3 Diploma, and some companies may ask for a period of commercial experience from their applicants. Many of these companies personally train their employees in-house, and then distribute them to cruise ships. Companies such as this often come into institutions such as colleges, looking to recruit new, aspiring therapists.

For the majority of people, travelling on a cruise ship is a luxury option. Cruise ships offer hotel quality service, whilst out on the open water. Customers will often be at sea for weeks at a time, and therefore an integral part of this service involves hiring a team of on-board hairdressers, makeup artists and beauty therapists, to ensure that customers have a full range of services at their disposal. As a cruise ship therapist, as you would anywhere else in the world, it is your job to make the customers and travellers feel as good as they possibly can, both physically and mentally. If you are someone who loves to travel, loves helping and meeting new people on a regular basis, then this could be a perfect position for you.

As a cruise ship therapist, you would work on board a ship, providing luxury beauty treatments and services to clients. These could range from anything to massages, pedicures, electrolysis or facial treatments. There are many misconceptions about working on board a cruise ship. Many people see it as a glamorous, easy option, which will get them a free trip around the world. This is certainly not the case. Working on board a cruise ship is extremely hard work. Whereas in a local salon, you might have several breaks a day, or periods where you aren't performing physical treatments; on a cruise ship, particularly amongst wealthy cliental, you will be working non-stop almost every day. The cliental will have higher expectations, and you will have to perform to these expectations, on a constant basis. While all your expenses and accommodation will be paid for, and you will get to visit many different and exotic areas of the world, you will have to work hard to earn these privileges. You will be expected to sell and promote products at an extremely high rate, and there will be set rules and regulations as to what activities you can take part in whilst on board the ship. The pay for working on a cruise ship can also vary. Since your food and accommodation are already paid for, you will be making similar to minimum wage, for around 12 hours work per day, and will rely heavily on tips. If you are considering working on a cruise ship, you also need to make sure that you are someone who is comfortable with spending long periods away from home, being on the water for weeks at a time and working for 6 or 7 days a week. Most therapists are hired on a non obligatory, 6 month basis, and therefore this is not a job with great security. You will likely share a room with fellow crew members, and there will be a communal area for luxuries such as television and entertainment.

As a cruise ship therapist, your duties will include:

- Reporting to your spa manager/assistant manager.

- Providing various types of massage, skin care and luxury treatment.

- Applying day and night makeup, eyelash tinting, eyebrow waxing and HD Brow treatment.

- Identifying wellness concerns and potential skin issues, particularly important as customers are on a boat for weeks at a time.

- Maintaining personal appearance at all times in order to keep with company values and expectations.

- Promoting and selling company products to customers.

Application and Interview

If you do decide to work on a cruise ship, there are a number of options available to you. Applying for jobs on a cruise ship, in today's market, is as simple as performing a quick Google search. You can also search for 'the big 3', Royal Caribbean, Carnival or Norwegian Cruise lines, and use their website to look for vacancies. Due to the workload and turnover of the role, there are thousands of these positions available every year. While it is a competitive market, if you are someone with the right qualities then you stand a great chance of being hired. There are also cruise ship recruitment agencies available, whom you can contact to try and increase your chances of getting an interview.

When filling in your application form, and cover letter, make sure you tailor your qualities to match what the role is looking for. The ordinary response, for most people, would be to highlight their sense of adventure and desire to travel the world. You should concentrate on your hard work ethic, ability to sell products at a constant rate, and an understanding of what the role will entail. Make sure the company sees you as someone who will have no issue with travelling and being away from home for long periods of time. If you are successful, you will be invited to an interview with the salon manager/the person you will be working under, during your time on the ship.

Questions for a cruise ship interview may include any of the following:

Why have you chosen to work on a ship, instead of in a regular salon?

How much do you know about our company?

Do you understand how the workload differs to a salon?

Have you ever sailed, or had experience working on a ship in the past?

What do you think you can bring to our on board salon?

When answering all of these questions, make sure you take into account the information we have given you, about how working on board a ship is not 'just a travel experience', but is a disciplined and hard-working role that requires maximum commitment from the employee.

With all this in mind, we have provided you with a list of our top tips, for working as a cruise ship therapist. We hope you find them useful.

- **Be prepared to work hard.** You will be expected to work an absolute minimum of 5 days a week, most of these days consisting of 10 hours or more.

- **Make sure you are comfortable travelling.** If you are not someone who is happy being away from home, or being cut off from the outside world for long periods of time, this is not the job for you.

- **Don't expect to live like one of the passengers.** As we have explained, you will be given very little leisure time as an employee on board a cruise ship. The food you eat, the quarters you sleep in and the entertainment services you will be provided, will also not be of the same quality. During your days off, you are free to explore the ship, or wherever the ship has landed, but any money you spend will be completely your own.

- **Make a contingency plan.** The non-committal nature of this job means that often, employees are left in the lurch when the liner or salon cuts their contract. You should always have a backup plan in place, in the event of this happening.

CHAPTER 10

Conclusion

There are so many different options available for aspiring therapists, that sometimes deciding which option to take can be a confusing and difficult process. We really hope that this guide has made your decision easier, and given you a clearer perspective on what the next step in your career path should be. Regardless of whether you decide to work in a salon, independently or on a cruise ship, remember the key attributes that will allow you to succeed within the beauty industry. These are:

- **A social and friendly personality.** You must be a warm and reassuring figure, with whom your clients can relate. Remember that you are not just a physical therapist, but someone that clients can talk and open up to. Be prepared to deal with clients who are not always friendly, or who are extremely fussy and particular with their demands. You must be someone who can act pleasantly even towards people you may not necessarily like.

- **Be willing to learn and adapt.** The industry is constantly changing and updating its methods, and therefore so must you. You will learn new treatment methods every year, and must be ready and willing to put these into practice. Stay up to date by using the internet to research upcoming treatments, and visiting trade and market shows.

- **Take care of your own appearance.** While you won't get hired based on your looks, your general appearance will certainly be taken into account. Salon owners will be looking to hire individuals who reflect their business values, and represent these to the customer. Chipped nails or unwashed hair will tell the salon that you aren't someone who cares about your appearance, and therefore won't care about the customers. Make sure you are in pristine condition before heading off to work each day.

- **Be organised.** Remember that being a beauty therapist is almost never a 9-5 job. If you work in a salon, you'll have to come in early, and finish later. If you work independently, you'll have to spend some of your evenings working on promotion and preparing for the next day, and if you work on a cruise ship, you can expect almost no leisure time at all. All of this means that as a therapist, you have to manage your time efficiently. You must be prepared to deal with setbacks that cut into your break-time, and to work for as long as necessary to ensure client satisfaction.

When researching for this book, we took the time to interview several therapists within the field. We asked them about their experiences, how much they enjoy the role and what advice they would give to any aspiring therapists. As our final gift to you, we have provided all of the results to this below. We hope you find it useful.

Questionnaire Results

What is your job?

Jo: *I lecture in beauty at my local college.*

Wendy: *I'm the co-owner of a salon, and lecture at college.*

Samantha: *I'm the Head of Hair and Beauty at a general further education college.*

How long have you worked as a beautician?

Jo: *31 years*

Wendy: *26 years*

Samantha: *30 years*

Did you always want to be a beauty therapist?

Jo: *Yes, I think I did, either that or an interior designer, as I love to paint and decorate things.*

Wendy: *My original goal was to be a system analyst, but when that didn't materialise, I took beauty instead.*

Samantha: *Yes, right from the careers interview at my school.*

Why did you decide to open your own salon? Was there any particular inspiration, or a story behind your decision?

Wendy: I started helping with training at the salon I co-own, then took the place of another partner when she decided to leave.

How have you found it being the boss?

Wendy: Usually it's good, especially since there are two of us in control. Sometimes it can be stressful when the finances are tight.

Samantha: Tough. Really tough at times. You have to make unpopular decisions and some days you feel like you have only just dealt with problems. However, when things go well and your team are happy, you know you played a role in that, and it is a rewarding feeling.

Have you ever worked independently, or always as part of a team/salon? Can you think of any advantages or disadvantages to working independently?

Jo: Always as part of a team, which I've been happy with as I am a great team player.

Samantha: Both. On your own can be lonely, especially when things are not going too well, but it is peaceful and you can achieve quite a large amount of work with very little distraction. I have worked in several teams, you can pull together when times are tough and the workload can be shared, but it is distracting when team members don't pull their weight. I really like my current job where I get to work in a team but also complete a lot of work on my own. The beauty industry is perfect for that, you can work for a large salon/spa but spend a large amount of time on your own with clients.

How does the role benefit you personally?

Jo: I really get along with the people I work with, and often see them outside of work. The holidays are also a huge benefit.

Wendy: It is a personable job by nature, you have lots of really pleasant interactions and great conversations, and you learn a lot from the public! It can be relaxing to perform certain treatments and you quickly learn how to handle people, making them feel at ease. This has really helped me in my management role.

What are your normal working hours?

Jo: 09:00-18:00, including preparing paperwork for the next day.

Wendy: 08:00-19:00 most weekdays, with some Saturdays and Sundays.

Samantha: 08:00-19:00 most weekdays, with some Saturdays and Sundays.

What is your favourite, and least favourite treatment to give?

Jo: My favourite treatment to perform is facials, my least favourite is a pedicure.

Wendy: I like giving facials and massage, my least favourite would be pedicures or manicures.

Samantha: My favourite is a facial, I love making someone's skin look and feel better, and the same applies to my own face!

What are the top 3 things about working in beauty?

Wendy: My top three things about working in beauty are: Helping clients to relax and feel less stressed, making a difference to clients' looks and mental well-being, and meeting new people.

Samantha: My favourite things about working in the beauty industry are: There is always something new to learn, you get to work with luxurious brands and products, and the job is so sociable.

What are the worst 3 things about working in beauty?

Wendy: My worst three things about working in beauty would be: Standing for long periods of time, RSI (repetitive strain injury) and the unsociable hours.

Samantha: The worst three things about working in the industry are: Standing on your feet all day, the lack of breaks you get during a busy day at the salon, and the fact that clients are often late, putting you behind schedule and causing other customers to be unhappy when their treatment is delayed.

What is the number 1 quality required to work within the beauty industry?

Jo: A cheerful personality.

Wendy: You have to get along with, and like people.

Samantha: You need to be able to provide great customer service.

How difficult do you find it if you have to perform a treatment on a client who isn't clean, or smells bad? Can you give any advice for dealing with these situations?

Jo: It's very unpleasant, luckily it's only happened to me a couple of times. After a while you get used to it though.

Samantha: It's a challenge. It really depends on whether it will affect the treatment or not. I was once waxing a client, whose skin was so dirty (she had been at a music festival) that I couldn't complete the treatment, it would have been too unhygienic. You have to make a judgement each time. It doesn't happen very often and you can always invite your client to have a relaxing shower before their massage.

What is the biggest lesson you have learned, and the biggest problem you have had to overcome?

Jo: The biggest lesson I have learned, is to always double-check what clients want.

Wendy: During my time in this industry, I have learned to engage in conversation and to listen to people.

Samantha: Don't make assumptions about anybody! People can be deceptive and surprise you, in a good way. The biggest problem I have had to overcome is persuading young people to fulfil their potential. So many students give up too easily. Studying is hard, work is hard and you only get out what you put in.

When conducting college interviews, what are the qualities you most look for in a candidate? Likewise, if interviewing someone for a salon job, what qualities do you look for?

Jo: I look for a candidate with the ability to converse, who has an interest in the industry.

Wendy: The best candidates are well presented, polite and ask lots of questions at the end. I want someone who is interested in working within the business, and my salon.

Samantha: I look for candidates who are personable and friendly, can give examples of what they have achieved, have a sensitive and caring manner and display ambition and drive towards their career.

What is your advice for any future, aspiring beauty therapists?

Jo: It's very hard work, but if you are keen then don't limit your expectations to 'just working in a salon'. Travel and expand on your experiences.

Wendy: Aim high! You have a really interesting career ahead of you.

Samantha: It's a very demanding, hectic job, but lovely and rewarding at times too. It's great meeting new people and gaining trust with clients. There are much worse jobs in the world; I love what I do!

Useful Resources

Training and Qualifications

British Association of Beauty Therapy and Cosmetology (BABTAC).
http://www.babtac.com

Confederation of International Beauty Therapy and Cosmetology (CIBTAC).
http://www.cibtac.com

VTCT examination awarding body
http://www.vtct.org.uk

Insurance Providers

The Beauty Guild: http://www.beautyguild.com

Salon Saver: http://www.salonsaver.co.uk

Professional Beauty: http://www.professionalbeauty.co.uk/

ABT Insurance: http://abtinsurance.co.uk/

Websites and Magazines

Salon Geek: http://www.salongeek.com

Professional Beauty Magazine:
http://www.professionalbeauty.co.uk

BABTAC Vitality: http://www.babtac.com/vitality-magazine/

Further Information

How2become also offers the below related titles:

- *How to Become a Mobile Hairdresser*
- *How to Become a Nail Technician*
- *How to Become a Massage Therapist*

Visit https://www.how2become.com/ to find out more.